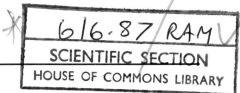
# POSTVIRAL FATIGUE
# SYNDROME

## The saga of Royal Free disease

### ERRATA

1. The first paragraph on page 24 should appear on page 21. It refers to the Athens outbreak.
2. The final sentence of the first paragraph on page 49 should read: Is it not possible that both these mechanisms may play a part in causing relapse and, in so many cases, permanent disability?

Further copies available from the
Myalgic Encephalomyelitis Association
The Association
P.O. Box 8
Stanford le Hope
Essex SS17 8EX

*Front cover illustration:* Electron
micrograph of an enveloped herpes
virus, showing the core, with
capsomeres, and the outer envelope.
x200,000. Courtesy of Heather
Davies, Clinical Research Centre,
Harrow.

# POSTVIRAL FATIGUE SYNDROME

# SYNDROME

## The saga of Royal Free disease

## A. Melvin Ramsay MA MD

Honorary Consultant Physician in Infectious Diseases,
Royal Free Hospital

Produced by Gower Medical Publishing, London
for the Myalgic Encephalomyelitis Association

ISBN: 0 906923 96 4

Editor: Marion Jowett
Designer: Christopher Inns

Typeset by TNR Productions Ltd, London.

Printed in Great Britain by Butler & Tanner Ltd.

# FOREWORD

The time is propitious for the publication of an authoritative account of that mysterious illness, formerly known as Royal Free, Akureyri or Iceland disease, epidemic vegetative neuritis or epidemic neuromyasthenia, and now called myalgic encephalomyelitis. With hindsight, it is easy to see why a whole variety of hypotheses has been put forward to explain its occurrence and why the puzzled clinician, brought up in the rigid discipline of 'no physical signs – no disease', dismissed the unfortunate sufferer as hysterical.

Dr Melvin Ramsay knows the whole saga: he was one of the pioneers involved in the investigation of the first outbreak, he realized that the disease was organic and he has made a life-time study of its protean manifestations. The disease follows viral infections, and laboratories on each side of the Atlantic have now provided convincing evidence that these patients do have histological, electrophysiological and immunological abnormalities. Scientists have recently come to the aid of Dr Ramsay in identifying the many complications, and especially the subtle abnormalities in cellular function, which may be associated with chronic viral illnesses.

Myalgic encephalomyelitis, dismissed so summarily a few years ago as a purely hysterical illness, may prove to be the epitome of a new type of disease, dependent on the propensity of viruses to persist in the most highly differentiated cells of the body. The many technical advances in immunology, biochemistry, molecular biology and genetics can be expected to confirm Dr Ramsay's original hypothesis. When this happens, a rational mode of therapy can at last be proposed and a host of patients will owe him a great debt of gratitude.

P.O. Behan, MD, FRCP, FACP
*Consultant Neurologist,*
*Reader in Neurology,*
*Glasgow University*

# ACKNOWLEDGEMENTS

I should like to express my gratitude to the members of the Study Group who, since the symposium in 1978, have met at frequent intervals to discuss the fostering of research. I am especially indebted to Dr Betty Scott who, following the Finchley outbreak, collaborated with me in the clinical assessment of cases from all parts of the United Kingdom and from abroad and to Dr Gordon Parish who has given me invaluable advice and assistance based on his exhaustive and searching study of the literature which has accrued on the subject. I am greatly indebted to Dr P.O. Behan for his appreciation of my work expressed in the foreword and for his help in respect of recent publications. I am equally indebted to Dr W.H. Lyle for his very generous assistance in obtaining reprints of important articles and to Professor James Mowbray for his encouragement and advice.

# CONTENTS

# NOMENCLATURE

The syndrome to which Royal Free disease belongs is one that follows an infectious disease process which is probably caused by a virus, although no specific aetiological agent has been identified. An outbreak which occurred in Iceland in 1948–49 was named both 'Iceland disease' and 'Akureyri disease' after the name of the town in which it first appeared. The use of such names is to be regretted since it tends to limit the disease to particular geographical sites and obscures the fact that the condition is to be found worldwide. I would strongly recommend that such terms be discarded. The leader writer in the *Lancet* (1956), under the title 'A New Clinical Entity?', suggested that a suitable term might be 'benign myalgic encephalo-myelitis'. The word 'benign' can only be justified on the grounds that there is no mortality from the disease and Dr Sigurdsson (1956) registered strong objections to its use as it was 'certainly not benign in other respects'. I have no doubt that many victims who are permanently incapacitated would readily agree. I therefore suggest that the term 'epidemic myalgic encephalomyelitis', put forward by a leader writer in the *British Medical Journal* in 1978, is preferable. Colloquially we tend to refer to it as 'ME' and this is certainly suitable for the many sporadic cases which are endemic and occur unrelated to any epidemic. In America the term 'epidemic neuro-myasthenia' was introduced to describe the neuritic and muscle abnormalities and was adopted by the physicians who reported the outbreak at the Great Ormond Street Hospital in 1970 because the neurological findings were sparse. The term was used in the symposium held at the Royal Society of Medicine in 1978, in deference to several American colleagues who read papers. A further term, 'postviral fatigue syndrome', has been coined and this has been accepted on both sides of the Atlantic, thus avoiding the confusion which arises from different names for the same disease.

For the purposes of this narrative, I propose to use the term ME, with which we have all been familiar for so many years past.

# 1

## The events of the momentous year 1955

### Synopsis

This chapter comprises: a very full account of the outbreak in the Royal Free Hospital, London, between July 13 and November 24; an account of a series of sporadic cases which occurred over a large area of North-West London preceding and giving rise to the outbreak within the hospital and persisting for nearly three years; an account of an outbreak in the village of Dalston in Cumbria, commencing in February of that year and spreading to the north east in July with cases in the area of Durham and other towns; and, finally, an account of a similar outbreak in Addington Hospital, Durban, South Africa, also commencing in February 1955.

## An outbreak of encephalomyelitis in the Royal Free Hospital

On July 13th 1955 a resident doctor and a ward sister on the staff of the Royal Free Hospital were admitted to the wards with an obscure illness. By July 25th more than 70 members of the staff were similarly affected and it was plain that there was in the hospital an epidemic of a highly infectious nature producing, among other things, manifestations in the central nervous system. Because of the threat to the health of patients and because of the large number of nurses involved, the hospital closed on that date and remained closed until October 5th. By that time the epidemic was almost over although sporadic cases appeared up to November 24th.

Between July 13th and November 24th, 292 members of the medical, nursing, auxiliary medical, ancillary and administrative staff were affected by the illness and of these, 255 were admitted to hospital; 37 nurses were looked after at home or admitted to other hospitals from their home. It is remarkable that, although the hospital was full at the time of the epidemic, only 12 patients who were already there developed the disease.

These are the opening two paragraphs of the report on the outbreak published in the *British Medical Journal* of October 19, 1957, by the medical staff of the hospital who were concerned with the care of these patients. The clinical picture which they described was based on the findings in two hundred of these cases in which the diagnosis seemed certain and in which the records were complete. No analysis was made of the ninety-two cases which were omitted and, with the gift of hindsight, this omission was to prove singularly unfortunate since they contained many instances of nurses who had succumbed to panic at the rapidity with which their friends and colleagues were going down with a 'mystery illness'. As a result of this, at a later date, Drs McEvedy and Beard were presented with abundant material for their hypothesis of 'mass hysteria' (see Chapter 4).

The earliest symptoms were malaise and headache, frequently associated with disproportionate depression and emotional lability. Early symptoms fluctuated markedly, often disappearing for a day or two only to return **more severely**. A mild sore throat was usual; headache, frontal or occipital, though often transient, could be persistent and severe; and nausea with anorexia was frequent. Transient abdominal pain, vomiting and diarrhoea were less common. In a few cases the fully developed picture did not manifest until the second or third week. This consisted of pain in the neck, back or limbs and of dizziness. The pain was out of proportion to the general constitutional disturbance and was sometimes present when fever was absent. It was usually confined to one limb, one side of the body or to both legs and, as with other symptoms, pain showed marked variation from day to day or even from one part of the day to another. Pain below both rib margins was common and at times the severity of these pains was such as to require the strongest analgesics for their control. Dizziness, usually a transient feeling of imbalance on sudden movement but in some a true vertigo, characterized the disease in the early stages. Sometimes the vertigo was very marked, being readily induced by slight movement of the head.

During the second and third weeks many of the patients became more severely ill. In addition to the intensification of the earlier symptoms, particularly of the pain, prostration and vertigo, other neurological symptoms and signs developed. One hundred and forty-eight patients out of the two hundred (74%) showed objective evidence of involvement of the central nervous system and the neurological manifestations formed a characteristic picture that distinguishes this disease from other infections of the nervous system. There was heavy involvement of the cranial nerves. Transient

2

blurring of near vision, probably due to weakness of the ciliary muscle, was encountered; the pupils were at times unequal and were sometimes defective in reaction to light and on accommodation. Weakness of the external muscles of the eye was common and sometimes both sides were affected. Paralysis of the face occurred in just under 20% of cases and occasionally both sides were affected. Vertigo could persist and become very severe, and could be associated with tinnitus and nystagmus. Paralysis of swallowing occurred in eleven patients and two of these required tube-feeding.

The limbs and trunk were involved in almost all cases in which the nervous system was involved. Motor weakness was more common than sensory disturbance. Initially the weakness was accompanied by loss of tone and could be associated with severe and painful muscle spasms that often occurred in limbs in which there was clear objective evidence of sensory disturbance. The slightest attempt at active or passive movement could invoke extreme pain. Loss of power in the affected limbs was more marked in the lower, rather than the upper, muscles and in some cases the paralysis was complete. Sometimes early on, but more commonly during recovery from weakness, a peculiar jerking was noted in a limb on voluntary movement. This is considered to be a distinctive and characteristic feature of nerve involvement in this form of encephalomyelitis.

In addition to spasm, irritative phenomena such as twitching and fasciculation (rippling of muscle seen under the skin) were noted and all of these became more pronounced when the patient was disturbed by physical movement or nursing treatment. Bladder dysfunction occurred in one quarter of the patients and consisted of difficulty in micturition which could result in retention requiring tidal drainage for a few days.

Spontaneous pain was the commonest sensory manifestation and its part in the clinical picture cannot be overemphasized. It was usually felt diffusely throughout a weak limb and was associated with marked muscle tenderness. There could be extreme tenderness in the regions below the ribs and attempts at examination sometimes evoked resentment due to pain. Weakness and coarse tinglings chiefly in the limbs, were further sensory manifestations. Objective sensory loss was usually marked in the lower part of the limbs and this coincided with the motor weakness. In a number of patients there was a complete loss of sensation over one half of the body, although the face usually escaped.

The clinical impression was of a disease producing a diffuse

3

disorder of the nervous system with a combination of irritative and paralytic signs which were frequently transient. The most important evidence of the generalized infectious process was to be found in the involvement of other systems:

|  | % of cases |
|---|---|
| Posterior cervical glands enlarged | 79 |
| Anterior cervical glands enlarged | 52 |
| Axillary glands enlarged | 36.5 |
| Inguinal glands enlarged | 32.5 |
| Tenderness below rib margins | 32.5 |
| Neck rigidity | 11 |
| Epitrochlear glands enlarged | 10 |
| Liver edge palpable | 8.5 |
| Severe injection of the pharynx | 6 |
| Vesicles on pharynx | 6 |

Electromyograms carried out on twenty-eight patients confirmed that there was involvement of the motor unit at the level of the spinal cord. Intensive laboratory investigations failed to reveal the causal agent. This then was the 'event' which became known as 'Royal Free disease' and which has since attained notoriety as a suspected outbreak of 'mass hysteria', the context in which it occurred being either ignored or forgotten. It may be that the explosive nature of the outbreak and the failure to detect the causal agent, despite intensive investigations, are responsible for its being regarded as an isolated baffling episode. However, I find that there has been a general failure on the part of the profession to recognize that:

1. the outbreak in the hospital arose as a direct result of a nest of sporadic cases over a large area of North West London which had been present since the spring
2. an outbreak of infection of a very extensive nature had commenced in Dalston, Cumbria, in February 1955 and had spread to the north east of the country by July
3. an outbreak closely similar to that in the Royal Free Hospital had occurred in Addington Hospital, Durban, South Africa, in February of that momentous year.

4

## The outbreak in North West London, 1955–58

In May 1955 we found that we were admitting to the Infectious Diseases Department of the Royal Free Hospital at Hampstead cases which were frankly puzzling, although the degree of muscular weakness at first suggested a diagnosis of poliomyelitis. In 1955 we admitted sixteen such cases, in 1956 there were eighteen and in 1957 another nineteen. Together with a few cases early in 1958 this constituted an outbreak which had lasted almost three years. The initial features generally took the form of an upper respiratory tract infection with low-grade fever, sore throat, enlarged cervical glands or, less commonly, a gastrointestinal upset and, in five cases, acute vertigo. The patients then complained of persistent headache, sometimes both frontal and occipital and accentuated by movement, while intermittent attacks of vertigo could occur throughout the early period. In addition, patients complained of pain in the limbs, neck and back, paraesthesiae and visual phenomena in the form of blurring of vision, while actual diplopia was by no means an infrequent occurrence. Muscle cramps, spasms, twitchings and deep muscle tenderness were common but the **dominant feature was muscle fatigability**; following even a minimal degree of physical exertion there could be delays of three to five days before muscle power was restored. Lymphadenopathy, affecting mainly the posterior chain of the cervical glands, and exaggerated tendon reflexes were found in over 50% of cases. Impairment of sensation was present in 41% and presented as excessive sensitivity of the skin, usually corresponding with areas of deep muscle tenderness, interspersed with areas of hypoalgesia. Extensor plantar responses were found in 21% of cases and in two cases these persisted after discharge from hospital. We found nystagmus in 23% of cases and cranial nerve palsies in 10%. Evidence of involvement of the autonomic nervous system was present in most cases. This could take the form of orthostatic tachycardia [which Sotomayer (1969) pointed out does not occur in hysteria], coldness of the extremities and hypersensitivity to climatic change, and a ghastly facial pallor often first noticed by friends or relatives. A very common feature was bladder disturbance, a phenomenon reported by many observers. Frequency of micturition is a common legacy of these cases yet no evidence of infection of the urinary tract has ever been found, suggesting that weakness of the sphincter muscle could be the cause. A third component of the clinical picture of ME is cerebral involvement which usually takes the form of impairment of memory and powers of concentration, emotional lability and vivid dreams (often in colour) which tended to occur in persons who had had no previous experience of such phenomena. A complaint of hyperacusis (intolerance of loud noise) was by no means infrequent and this could alternate with periods of normal hearing or even deafness.

All the first eight and a large number of subsequent cases were submitted to electrophysiological investigations. These were carried out by Richardson (1956) and his findings were identical with those which he reported in the Royal Free Hospital outbreak. Electroencephalograms were carried out in five patients who had serious behaviour disorder: all were abnormal. At the early stage at which the examinations were made the changes were probably non-specific and possibly constitutional. However, Pampiglione, Harris & Kennedy (1978), at the Department of Electroencephalography in the Royal Free Hospital, demonstrated abnormalities in 38 patients even after a considerable period from the onset of the disease.

The first eight cases in this outbreak were described by the late Dr E. O'Sullivan and myself in the *Lancet* of May 26, 1956. They received very favourable comment in a leading article in the same issue and I have already commented on the suggestion made for the use of the term 'benign myalgic encephalomyelitis'. In the *Lancet* of December 14, 1957, I described thirty-four cases of this 'new entity'. These all conformed to the pattern described in the earlier publication. All cases, whether with or without neurological involvement, showed **proneness to fatigue after physical exertion** and by this time it was clear that this **could persist for weeks or months after the initial attack.** Most patients exhibited outbursts of irritability which proved very distressing to those who, previously of a calm and equable temperament, were fully aware of a change in disposition which no effort of will could control. At the symposium held at the Royal Society of Medicine in April 1978, I was able to present the records of fifty-three patients who were involved in this outbreak in North West London. At the same symposium Dr Nigel Compston reviewed in detail the events of the outbreak in the Royal Free Hospital and concluded that 'those of the medical staff of the hospital who witnessed the epidemic of 1955 were firmly of the opinion that they were dealing with an organic illness complicated by encephalomyelitis in which myalgia was a dominant feature. Objective evidence of brain stem and spinal cord involvement was observed.'

In 1978 I was able to report on the clinical and biochemical findings in ten patients with 'benign myalgic encephalomyelitis'.

This enquiry was carried out with the cooperation of Dr Alan Rundle, consultant pathologist at St Lawrence's Hospital, Caterham, and the results were published in the *Postgraduate Medical Journal* of December 1979 (see Tables 1 and 2). The investigation was based on blood levels of serum myoglobin and various enzymes and these showed a biochemical pattern closely similar to that found in Duchenne muscular dystrophy, though differing sharply in that we found no rise in creatine phosphokinase (CPK) levels in any of the patients. A difference in the molecular weights of myoglobin and CPK might afford an explanation for this. Whereas CPK is a relatively large molecule, with a molecular weight of 81 000, myoglobin has a molecular weight of 17 500. High levels of serum myoglobin, maintained in two successive estimations in all ten cases, were clearly indicative of muscle damage. Moreover, the level of one of the enzymes (glutamic oxaloacetic transaminase) was raised in all ten cases; in two the elevation was gross. Fasting whole-blood levels of lactate, pyruvate and ATP were estimated in five cases. The ATP level was normal in all five. The serum pyruvate was significantly reduced in all five, but serum lactate was low in only one case.

| Case | Sex | Myoglobin 1st | Myoglobin 2nd | CPK | γ-GTP | GOT | GPT |
|------|-----|------|------|------|------|------|------|
| 1 | F | 48 | 38 | 12 | 23 | 80 | 14 |
| 2 | F | 62 | 44 | 12 | 11 | 40 | 7 |
| 3 | F | 125 | 106 | 17 | 15 | 36 | 11 |
| 4 | M | 175 | 125 | 12 | 21 | 37 | 8 |
| 5 | F | 280 | 185* | 17 | 13 | 37 | 6 |
| 6 | F | 240 | 112* | 17 | 8 | 20 | 42 |
| 7 | F | 330 | 370 | 37 | 31 | 224 | 56 |
| 8 | M | 140 | 235 | 37 | 508 | 31 | 10 |
| 9 | F | 840 | 70* | 25 | 13 | 21 | 12 |
| 10 | F | 175 | 134 | 25 | 16 | 24 | 18 |
| Normal values | F | 12–76 | | 0–50 | 4–18 | 0–12 | 0–12 |
| | M | 19–96 | | | 6–28 | | |

*Subjects in a recovery phase when second blood sample taken.

**Table 1** Serum myoglobin (μg/ml) and serum levels of creatine phosphokinase (CPK), γ-glutamylpeptidase (γ-GTP), glutamic oxaloacetic transaminase (GOT) and glutamic pyruvic transaminase (GPT), all in i.u./l, in ten ME patients.

7

| Case | Sex | Pyruvate | Lactate | ATP |
|------|-----|----------|---------|-----|
| 1 | M | 0.13 | 7.8 | 24.2 |
| 2 | M | 0.24 | 49.3 | 13.7 |
| 3 | F | 0.09 | 12.8 | 21.8 |
| 4 | F | 0.09 | 11.8 | 18.4 |
| 5 | F | 0.19 | 11.6 | 22.1 |
| Normal values | | 0.36–0.59 | 9–16 | 19–32 |

**Table 2** Fasting whole-blood levels in pyruvate, lactate and ATP (mg/100ml) in five ME cases.

In a survey of clinical enzymology, Wilkinson (1978) discussed the release of enzymes from cells. He concluded that 'intracellular energy content is important in the control of membrane permeability' and gave as examples 'loss of enzymes from a series of insults such as anoxia, deprivation of glucose, high potassium concentrations, high-energy phosphate, and metabolic inhibitors such as both rat muscle and human erythrocytes'. Therefore, if the aetiological factor in ME impairs the permeability of the muscle cell membrane as a result of changes in the intracellular energy content, this could be followed by a differential loss of intracellular proteins.

### The outbreak in Dalston, Cumbria

Although it was unknown to us at the time of the North West London and Royal Free Hospital outbreaks, an extensive outbreak had commenced in the villages of Dalston, Orton and Thursby in February 1955 and this was fully reported by the general practitioner concerned, Dr A.I. Wallis (1955, 1957). The first case was recorded in a male adult and by the beginning of February there was an extensive epidemic in the primary-school children, the main spread to adults taking place in March and April. The epidemic continued until July by which time two hundred and thirty-three cases had been reported out of the practice population of one thousand six hundred and seventy-five children, an incidence of 14%. The male:female ratio was 1:1. Twenty children boarded at the Carlisle Corporation Home in Dalston, mainly boys aged 5–15 years, were all affected. Secondary attacks in contacts occurred in several families after a primary host relapsed, suggesting that the patient had again become infectious. The possibility of glandular fever was considered but the

Paul–Bunnell test was consistently negative. The onset was abrupt after an incubation period of 5–7 days but some of the adults had a delayed onset, with the illness reaching its maximum after more than six weeks. Neurological symptoms occurred in 60% of the patients but the objective signs were mild. There were lesions of the ulnar nerve in eight patients. Non-specific abnormalities were noted in the EEGs in fifteen of the twenty-three patients tested. Virus investigations proved negative.

The characteristic features of the Dalston epidemic are most important and are set out in detail:

1. a systemic illness with relatively low fever or subnormal temperatures in delayed-onset cases and tenderness over enlarged glands, liver and/or spleen
2. marked muscle fatigability
3. mental changes, such as impairment of memory, changes in mood with behaviour changes in children, sleep disorders, irritability or depression
4. involvement of the autonomic system resulting in orthostatic tachycardia, coldness of the extremities, episodes of sweating or profound pallor, sluggish pupils, constipation and frequency of micturition, possibly as a result of a lesion of the hypothalamus
5. diffuse and variable involvement of the central nervous system, leading to ataxia, weakness and/or sensory changes in a limb, nerve root or a peripheral nerve such as the ulnar
6. muscle pain, tenderness and myalgia
7. recurrence in about 20% of patients over a period of several years.

By July 1955 the disease had spread eastwards to County Durham where the senior registrar in the electrodiagnostic clinic encountered a dramatic increase in the number of cases of lower motor neuron lesions, particularly ulnar nerve palsies, and of motor weakness of an unusual type affecting the shoulder girdle and legs. In August he himself was confined to bed with what was thought to be viral hepatitis without jaundice as there were similar cases in the district. When he was allowed to get up he noticed weakness of his legs which increased on walking. An attempt to return to work was followed by a more severe illness in October with a pyrexia up to 100.4°F (*c*.38°C) lasting several weeks. Although he returned to part-time work in January 1956 he relapsed the following summer. I saw him with Dr A.T. Richardson and we found that he had a marked right foot-drop. We diagnosed him as a case of ME. His history is of great interest as it shows the insidious-onset form of the disease and the type of course with severe relapses (in his case every three or four years) with periods of relatively good health in between. However, in the last few years his disability has become persistent as the result of repeated milder relapses.

## The outbreak in Addington Hospital, Durban

The remaining event of the year 1955 was an outbreak of infectious disease among the staff of Addington Hospital, Durban, in February 1955 and it is fitting to conclude this chapter with a brief account of the clinical features. It was reported by Hill, Cheetham & Wallace in 1959 and was an example of an outbreak which occurred while a recognized poliomyelitis epidemic was in progress and where the earlier cases were thought to be instances of that condition.

The disease struck with dramatic suddenness and within a week fifty-nine nurses became ill. In the next few weeks more nurses were affected, bringing the total to ninety-eight. There was no spread to other hospital personnel or to patients, thus lending support to the suggestion that some toxic substance was responsible for the outbreak. At first the disease was confined to nurses living within the hospital but later many of those who lived outside were affected. Then sporadic cases began to come in from the city and this, together with the failure to incriminate any known toxin, supported the theory of a disease of infectious origin. Indeed it soon became apparent that the hospital outbreak was an episode in an infection which had been occurring among the general population for some weeks or perhaps months and which had been unrecognized until it broke out with explosive force among the nurses. The similarity to the relationship between the outbreak in North West London and the outbreak among staff of the Royal Free Hospital is unmistakable.

The prodromal phase of the illness presented with severe occipital headache for up to fourteen days preceding the onset of the acute phase. The headache was usually accompanied by extreme lassitude, sore throat, painful or burning eyes, coryza and in some cases nausea, vomiting and diarrhoea with severe backache. The acute phase was ushered in by sudden weakness of the back and abdominal muscles and a feeling of heaviness in one or both extremities. Paraesthesiae or severe pain in the affected limb was common. Paresis was present in at least one extremity and attempts to exercise increased the weakness. The convalescent phase was variable; it could be short but in the majority it persisted for one to three months and tended to recur on return to duty. Relapses were identical with the initial onset and the disablement continued for six to nine months and then either resolved or persisted as a lack of endurance in the muscles originally involved. Eleven patients were still disabled after three years and ten of these have been invalided out of the service. The remaining one, a senior sister, has returned to duty with a permanent foot-drop. It was found that relapses of considerable severity continued to occur and while this usually involved the same muscles as in the original attack, sometimes other muscles were involved, even after an interval of many weeks. Most of the nurses exhibited inability to concentrate, defective memory, persistent drowsiness and emotional lability. Personality changes were evident in many and this was noted by friends or relatives. Mood changes which had not previously existed became evident.

I have set out the features of these outbreaks in some detail in order to establish that:

1. the outbreak in the Royal Free Hospital cannot be considered in isolation since the nidus of infection had been present in North West London for some time
2. another nidus of infection was present in Dalston from the very early part of the year and this spread to North-East England by midsummer
3. a similar outbreak occurred in Durban, 6000 miles away, and corresponded closely in that the nidus of infection was present in the general population before it exploded among hospital staff.

These outbreaks of infectious disease followed a classical pattern and left a legacy of many cases with permanent physical incapacity which in Durban rendered ten nurses unable to continue with their profession. The most important point is that **marked muscle fatigability** was the dominant clinical feature in all these outbreaks.

11

# 2

## Notes on other recorded outbreaks

### Synopsis
Up to the present time fifty-two outbreaks of this type of infection have been recorded from various parts of the world. Brief summaries of eighteen of these are presented here in order to establish the close similarity between them in respect of clinical features, particularly the presence of muscle fatigability in all, as well as the long legacy of physical incapacity which followed in very many cases.

### Los Angeles, 1934

In 1934 an epidemic of what was at first considered to be poliomyelitis occurred in Los Angeles. Indeed a number of outbreaks occurred in institutions with features which differed from those usually associated with poliomyelitis. The most important outbreak involved one hundred and ninety-eight members of the medical and nursing staff of Los Angeles County General Hospital. The main features of the illness were described by Gilliam (1938) who found that although the initial symptoms were similar to poliomyelitis, and localized muscle weakness occurred in 80% of cases, the severe degree of muscle wasting which is an invariable feature of poliomyelitis did not occur. Moreover, muscle pain and tenderness together with sensory symptoms persisted far longer than would be expected in poliomyelitis. Loss of concentration and lapses of memory, sleep disturbances and emotional lability with hysterical episodes were features of the disease and **fatigue on walking short distances** was a prominent feature. Recurrence of both systemic and neurological symptoms were frequent and some cases were more disabled by the recurrence than by the original illness. There was no mortality but morbidity was high; indeed 55% of the staff were still off duty six months after the peak of the epidemic.

Wilson & Walker (1936) stated that

vaso-motor and trophic disturbances were almost constant findings among the adult patients. Excessive sweating or

12

abnormal dryness of the skin of the extremities, together with coldness and cyanosis, were the phenomena usually observed. In the cases of more severe involvement, exfoliation of the skin of the affected extremities occurred, followed by glossy atrophy of the skin and atrophy of the subcutaneous tissue. Hypertrichosis and brittleness of the nails, with retardation or acceleration of growth were noted. It was the impression of many observers that a generalised disturbance of vaso-motor control occurred in these patients, which best explained the emotional instability and the exacerbations of the symptoms described later.

Between 1948 and 1952 Marinacci & Von Hagen (reported in 1965) examined twenty-one of the cases (that is, about 10%) and found that all had residual muscle pain, fatigue and mental changes. They found similar changes in three hundred cases of epidemic neuromyasthenia seen between 1948 and 1965 and observed that recurrences could still occur after seven years of normal health. They concluded that the disease was spread by personal contact with cases or carriers and that the illness may have been a modification of the prevailing illness, namely poliomyelitis, or may have been due to a coincidental infection of the central nervous system of which the cause remained unknown. To that I can only say that muscle weakness without resultant wasting of muscle cannot be poliomyelitis; indeed, the electromyogram which the authors mentioned showed no evidence of damage to the lower motor neuron and that in itself excludes poliomyelitis. Hysteria was recognized as a component of the illness but only a few cases were considered to be psychogenic.

Sporadic cases of the infection continued to appear in Los Angeles up to 1965. The outbreak in the Royal Free Hospital in 1955 was an almost exact replica of the outbreak in Los Angeles.

### Switzerland, 1937
Of nine hundred and thirty officers and men stationed at Erstfeld, Switzerland, in July 1937, one hundred and thirty were affected with an unknown infection within the space of twelve days; one hundred and four of these had a systemic illness and sixteen had meningeal involvement (*Gsell, 1938*). The soldiers developed encephalomyelitis

13

with mild muscle weakness. Sweating and hyperaesthetic areas were common features. A further outbreak in the summer was recorded in a women's section of a cantonal hospital at Frohburg, involving twenty-eight patients and staff. A prolonged convalescent period ensued with relapses, marked muscle fatigue and autonomic disturbance. The involvement of the central nervous system was more than twice as frequent among the hospital cases as among the soldiers.

## Switzerland, 1939
In September 1939, eight hundred officers and men arrived at Degersheim from an area in which there was an epidemic of poliomyelitis; the ensuing outbreak was described by Gsell (1949) as 'abortive poliomyelitis'. During September and in early October there were seventy-three cases of epidemic neuromyasthenia, fifty-four of whom had the systemic illness, the remainder having neurological involvement. In most cases the illness was short but disturbances of the autonomic nervous system were frequent in the convalescent period and muscle fatigability persisted in a few cases for more than a year.

The involvement of entirely male communities in two of the Swiss outbreaks just described, together with the fact that the male:female ratios in both the Adelaide and Dalston outbreaks were reported to be 1:1, should be remembered when the high female incidence in most outbreaks is advanced as a point favouring the hypothesis of 'mass hysteria'. The female preponderance in many outbreaks may be explained by occupational hazard among nurses.

## District epidemic in Iceland, 1948–49
In the autumn of 1948 three cases of what was considered to be 'classical poliomyelitis' occurred in the district of Akureyri; one was in the town itself. Thereafter, the clinical picture of epidemic neuromyasthenia developed and the disease spread to other districts in December 1948 and January 1949 (*Sigurdssen* et al., *1950*). Students at the high school were heavily involved so there was a very high incidence in the 15–19 age group. The systemic form of the illness occurred in 70% of patients with characteristic low-grade fever, muscle tenderness and marked lassitude. The remaining 30% had muscle weakness with pyrexia frequently over 100.4°F ($c.38$°C). Ulnar and shoulder girdle neuritis as well as radiculitis involving the T1, L5 and S1 nerve roots were described. Mental changes with hysterical episodes were observed. Multiple relapses occurred in

some patients with renewal of fever, muscle tenderness and weakness at a fresh site. Virus studies failed to show evidence of infection with poliomyelitis, Coxsackie or known encephalomyelitis viruses.

Now follows the really important feature of the Iceland outbreaks. In 1955 Kjartan Gudmundsson, a neurologist, re-examined thirty-nine patients affected in the 1948 epidemic and found that **of those more severely affected**, only 25% had recovered completely, while 52% had residual tenderness and **65% had objective neurological signs**. Many patients still complained of nervousness, **abnormal fatigability of muscles**, muscle pain, insomnia and loss of memory. **Of those mildly affected in 1948**, only 44% had fully recovered, while 50% had muscular tenderness and **19% had objective neurological signs** (*Sigurdsson & Gudmundsson, 1956*).

In the same year there was an epidemic of Type 1 poliomyelitis in Iceland and this spread around the coast, yet failed to become established at centres where epidemic neuromyasthenia occurred in 1948. It would therefore seem that the agent responsible for epidemic neuromyasthenia is able to inhibit the pathological effects of poliomyelitis infection.

## District epidemic in Adelaide, Australia, 1949–51

This was a further instance of an epidemic of poliomyelitis followed by cases presenting a different clinical picture. In contradistinction to the poliomyelitis cases, no abnormalities were found in the cerebrospinal fluid. The poliomyelitis epidemic commenced in May 1949 but it was not until August that cases of epidemic myalgic encephalomyelitis appeared and these continued to be seen until April 1951. By that time seven hundred cases had been admitted to hospital. The male:female ratio was 1:1. During the summer of 1950–51 the monthly incidence suggested that once the epidemic of ME had been triggered, its natural seasonal incidence paralleled that of poliomyelitis. Muscle weakness was slight but in some patients it appeared for the first time as late as three months after the onset of the initial symptoms (*Pellew, 1951; Pellew & Miles, 1955*).

No known virus was isolated in this epidemic but an agent was transmitted to monkeys and when the animals were killed, minute red spots were found along the sciatic nerves. Microscopically, infiltration of nerve roots with lymphocytes and monocytes was seen and some of the nerve fibres showed patchy damage in the myelin sheaths. This pathological picture of mild diffuse changes corresponded closely to what might have been expected from clinical observation of patients with neurological involvement in ME.

## District epidemic in New York State, 1950
In the autumn of 1950 an epidemic occurred in New York State which was diagnosed as 'abortive poliomyelitis'. White & Burtch (1954) recognized features such as muscular aches, sensory phenomena and nerve involvement throughout the course of the illness which were quite incompatible with a diagnosis of poliomyelitis, and they added, 'nor does the condition resemble any disease known to us'. The onset of the disease was acute in four cases and insidious in fifteen. The initial symptoms were of either an upper or a lower respiratory tract infection, but gastrointestinal symptoms also occurred. Tenderness of muscles was the most common feature and the muscles of the shoulder girdle were most frequently involved. Four patients complained of chest pain made worse on breathing; in the absence of a pleuritic friction rub it was concluded that the pain was the result of intercostal myalgia. Weakness affecting the limbs occurred at some time in the course of the illness and this persisted in two cases until re-examination sixteen months later. There was no muscle wasting as seen in poliomyelitis. Sensory symptoms were not infrequent and consisted of paraesthesiae and, less often, actual numbness. In two patients these symptoms involved the ulnar distribution to the arm and hand. In ten cases emotional lability was a 'remarkable feature' since it occurred in individuals of a known stoical disposition in whom such exhibitions were quite unusual. Re-examination of eight patients sixteen months after onset showed that not one was free of symptoms. Many patients reported that they tired more readily, particularly in the limbs in which the weakness had first occurred. All reported that they were more easily upset and more readily depressed than before they had been taken ill.

The authors concluded that the disease they had described had a striking resemblance to that described by Sigurdsson and others in Iceland. They considered that this was a new disease, distinct from poliomyelitis, and called it 'Iceland disease'.

## Middlesex Hospital, 1952
In the *Lancet* of November 20, 1954, Acheson reported the occurrence of an outbreak of infectious disease involving the central nervous system complicated by acute myalgia in fourteen nurses at the Middlesex Hospital. This outbreak was published on account of its unusual features and its resemblance to other atypical and

problematical epidemics reported in previous years. The characteristic feature of the outbreak was the association of severe muscular pains affecting the back, limbs, abdomen and chest with mild involvement of the central nervous system, the weight of the damage falling on the pyramidal tracts, the posterior columns and cranial nerves, rather than on the anterior horn cells. No case of poliomyelitis had been nursed in the hospital in the previous month nor had any cases of poliomyelitis or encephalomyelitis been notified from the adjacent boroughs.

This report is unique in that it contains the details of a case which in itself constitutes a complete refutation of the 'mass hysteria' hypothesis and I shall therefore quote it in full from the text:

Nurse A, aged 21, complained of headache and malaise, cramps in the legs and gripping pain in the abdomen with backache. Examination showed a temperature of 100°F and a patient who looked ill; there was pain on deviation of the eyes and a fine horizontal nystagmus. Minimal neck stiffness was noted. The day after admission she had severe headache, pain down the right side of the body, 'pins and needles' in the right hand and twitching in the right leg. During the day she developed difficulty in micturition followed by the sensation that things were 'sticking in her throat' and she had respiratory distress. She became drowsy and euphoric and meningism was more marked but her temperature had returned to normal. She showed nystagmus on looking to the right, poor movement of the soft palate, much tenderness in the right upper and lower limbs, mild paresis of the right shoulder muscles and moderate paresis of the flexors and extensors of the hand and of the dorsiflexors and plantar flexors of the right feet. The left side of the chest moved extremely poorly and, although the patient was not yet using her accessory muscles, she was taking about three breaths for each sentence. All the deep reflexes were depressed, the left more than the right. The right plantar response was extensor. In the next few days the deep reflexes of the right upper and lower limbs became exaggerated.

From this stage her recovery was uneventful except that on the fifth day of her illness she developed diplopia and later she was found to have diminished vibration sense in the right hand

and foot with absent position sense in the big toe. She was discharged 26 days after the start of her illness with numbness and slight weakness of the right foot and no position or vibration sense in the right big toe, minimal eversion of the right foot and an extensor right plantar response. These signs remained unchanged a year later.

## Epidemic neuromyasthenia in Washington, D.C., 1953
This outbreak was reported by Shelokov and his co-workers (1957) in the *New England Journal of Medicine*. In July 1953 a sharp outbreak of a disease thought to be poliomyelitis occurred in a private psychiatric hospital in Washington, D.C. Within a few days it became apparent that the epidemiological features and the course of the illness were not compatible with poliomyelitis but closely resembled the poliomyelitis-like outbreak which had occurred in Los Angeles in 1934. Search of the literature revealed that similar outbreaks had also occurred in Iceland, Australia, Denmark, England, South Africa and other parts of the world. On account of the epidemic no further nurses were taken for training during July and August but twenty-five new student nurses were admitted on August 31 and the first symptoms of a second outbreak were noted on September 18. Fifty persons were involved in these two outbreaks, twenty-six with confirmed paresis and twenty-four without paresis. As the latter group could have included cases influenced by anxiety and apprehension, the authors limited the description of cases to those who had paresis. In these a 'minor' illness preceded the paresis by four to six days. It was characterized by malaise, headache, general achiness and low-grade fever; when this phase exceeded five or six days, diarrhoea, nausea and vomiting became prominent. The onset of the 'major' illness was associated with aggravation of the prodromal symptoms followed by neck and spinal stiffness and a peculiar feeling of heaviness and numbness in a limb which became difficult to use; there was also **demonstrable diminution in muscle strength.** Temperatures seldom exceeded 101°F (*c*.38°C) but afternoon temperatures could be two or three degrees higher than the depressed morning ones. The authors described vasomotor disturbances consisting of both subjective and objective evidence of angiospasm in intermittent coldness and warmth of an affected extremity and cold clammy skin, becoming hot and flushed soon

afterwards. They also refer to **cutaneous sensory disturbances** of localized numbness and tinglings which did not conform to segmental distribution but were substantiated by changed response to pin-prick and light touch as either hypoalgesic (impaired) or hyperaesthetic (excessive). Twelve patients were re-examined in December 1953 and none reported feeling well. All had relapses and recrudescences at one time or another; some of the symptoms were precipitated by physical exertion, others by a change in ambient temperature or the onset of menstruation and these latter factors gave rise to sensations of unusual coldness in the extremities.

## Coventry 1953

'An illness resembling poliomyelitis observed in nurses' is the title of an article by Macrae & Galpine published in the *Lancet* in 1954. They reported that during the summer and autumn of 1953 some of the nurses in a Coventry hospital became ill with symptoms involving the central nervous system. Almost all were working in wards to which patients with poliomyelitis were being admitted and they were at first suspected of having that disease. The onset of their illness was insidious with mild sore throat, headache, backache, nausea, chills and lethargy. There was general muscle weakness in all but one of these patients. It was characterized by a feeling of aching in a limb, paraesthesiae in toes and slight cramps in the thighs; the patients found they tended to stumble when walking and the lower limbs became excessively fatigued. Paresis always affected one leg but could be present in three limbs and was associated with muscle tenderness and unsteadiness in response to effort. Areas of hyperaesthesia and hypoalgesia, with some loss of positional sense, were found. Difficulty in starting micturition was noted in four patients and one had to be catheterized for two days. Catheter specimens of urine were sterile and free of pus. Recovery took place within two months but undue aching and fatigue in the limbs persisted for much longer and several patients complained of difficulty in concentration. Most of the staff had multiple antibodies against poliomyelitis virus, indicating that they had a reasonable degree of immunity against that disease and that the cause of the outbreak was not the result of infection with that virus. The authors considered that the clinical findings were certainly indicative of an organic infective disorder.

In 1957, Galpine & Brady reported seven further cases which arose sporadically in the Coventry area in 1956. These gave clinical findings similar to those seen in 1953.

## An outbreak in Punta Gorda, Florida, 1956

An obscure epidemic illness occurred in a small Florida community in the spring of 1956 and was reported in full detail by Poskanzer and co-workers (1957). There were at least one hundred and fifty cases in a community of two thousand five hundred residents. The disease was more severe in females. No aetiological agent was discovered. The illness was characterized by fatigue, headache, neck pain, nausea and vomiting, paraesthesiae, aching muscular pain and variability in emotional status. It occurred among young and middle-aged patients and ran a prolonged relapsing course.

The severe long-term emotional and physical sequelae were so marked that twenty-one patients who presented with similar histories and who had no major intercurrent medical problems were selected for detailed clinical and laboratory study and were reassessed five months later by the same team of doctors. Seventeen of the twenty-one were female and patients ranged from 12 to 60 years of age. The onset was insidious and marked by increasing fatigue, headache, and pain in the neck, back and lower extremities. This was frequently accompanied by increased tension, depression and mental confusion. Fatigue, headache and neck pain were present in all the patients; the headache was severe, generalized, and dull and aching in character. In nineteen patients there was a memory defect for recent events with impaired ability in calculation or transient periods of mild confusion. Paraesthesiae taking the form of numbness and tingling in the extremities were a prominent feature and could have been related to hyperventilation in ten cases. Vertigo was also a prominent feature in the acute phase but less in evidence later. Visual disturbances including blurring of vision and diplopia were present in eleven cases. Temperatures exceeding $100°F$ ($37°C$) were only recorded in five patients.

The follow-up examination after five months showed that the course was an irregular one with periods of improvement interrupted by exacerbations of symptoms often related to physical exertion. The paucity of physical findings in relation to symptoms was striking. However, isolated areas of mild to moderate impairment of sensation to light touch or pin-prick were detected; these did not conform to the distribution of root or peripheral nerve zones. Focal muscle tenderness was noted at the time of the five-months review but these did not necessarily coincide with those detected at

20

the earlier examination. I made a precisely similar observation in my earlier writings on the subject (*Ramsay, 1978*). A positive Romberg test was found in five patients on their initial examination and in two on follow-up examination. Only one of the twenty-one patients was found to have been asymptomatic during the thirty days prior to his review examination.

Poskanzer and his co-workers found that a disproportionately high rate of illness was present in the medical and associated personnel and they considered that the multiple and protean symptoms reflected widespread disorders of function and that there were definite neurological disturbances, including impairment of memory, mental activity and sensation, as well as localized weakness and tenderness of muscle. They indicated that there was a strong similarity to outbreaks already reported in Iceland and Europe.

### An outbreak in a nurses' school in Athens, 1958
This outbreak was reported by Daikos and co-workers (1959). The previous year an obscure neurological illness involving twenty-seven cases had spread epidemically in the Queen Frederica School for Midwives. The patients were admitted to the University Department of Clinical Therapeutics. No patient or doctor in the Department of Obstetrics where the nurses had been working during the prodromal stage of the illness was affected. The prodromal phase was characterized by slight or severe muscular pains of two or three weeks' duration, accompanied by unsteady gait, numbness of the lower limbs, considerable weakness and malaise. When the disease was fully developed the pre-existing pains became more severe and in some this was accompanied by severe myalgia. The pains were located for the most part in the upper extremity, back or neck. Subjective sensory changes such as numbness, 'pins and needles' tinglings and a feeling of warmth in the affected limbs were prominent; anorexia, giddiness and occasionally diplopia were further features.

### Teachers' training college, Newcastle-upon-Tyne, 1959
A very interesting outbreak occurred in a teachers' training college in Newcastle-upon-Tyne in 1959 (*Pool* et al., *1960*). There were one hundred and twenty students in training and the college building was shared by a community of nuns who undertook the whole of the cooking for the college. Forty percent of the students were affected in the outbreak whereas only two of the nuns became ill. Presumably the sedentary nature of their lives protected them and this can be

considered in conjunction with the fact that only a very few of the patients in the Royal Free Hospital contracted the disease. Indeed a similar observation was made in the outbreak in Finchley described below.

**Outbreak in a convent in New York State, 1961**
This outbreak was described by Albrecht, Oliver & Poskanzer (1964). It occurred in a community of sixty-nine nuns over a seven-month period between July 1961 and January 1962. It took the form of an unusual type of illness characterized by a prolonged relapsing course. The symptoms were fatigue, muscle weakness, low-grade fever, nausea, headache and pain in the trunk or limbs, emotional lability, impairment of thinking, and paraesthesiae. Many patients complained that they had to give up their studies as they 'simply could not think'. Fifteen patients complained of distressing 'tightness' in the throat with a burning sensation below the sternum occurring continuously or on swallowing. Four patients complained of localized weakness in the hands, arms or legs and twelve of localized numbness, others of localized 'tinglings'. The authors commented that

physicians unfamiliar with the peculiar characteristics of previous epidemics . . . might easily dismiss these cases as hysteria . . . but that facile diagnosis is inadequate for reasons given by Acheson [1959] in his review of the subject as a whole . . . the mental symptoms of depression, emotional lability, impairment of memory and difficulty in concentration are consistent with organic brain disturbance and are different from the 'shallowness of affect' and 'belle indifference' of hysteria. In addition, symptoms and findings are consistent from outbreak to outbreak, in different countries, in different years, in different peoples.

In his letter to the *British Medical Journal* in 1970, Dr Poskanzer reminds us that in this outbreak he and his colleagues demonstrated a considerable increase in creatinuria and an increase in the creatine/creatinine ratio, suggesting an abnormality of muscle; these disappeared on recovery.

The authors also stressed the similarities of both the outbreaks in

New York State to that in Punta Gorda, Florida (see page 20).

Hypothermia as low as 95°F (35°C) was recorded in convalescent patients who complained of fatigue and feeling cold. Scott regarded three cases in young women admitted to hospital as a result of profound hypoglycaemia as a by no means infrequent feature of ME; all three made uneventful recoveries and she attributed this to the enforced rest in the early stages of the illness.

## Finchley outbreak, 1964–66
An outbreak of ME occurred in Finchley in 1964 and continued for two years. The cases were predominantly in the practice of Dr Betty Scott who reported in the *British Medical Journal* (1970) that she saw, in all, three hundred and seventy cases. Of these, twenty had been very seriously ill and had not been restored to their former state of health. In view of the assertion by Drs McEvedy & Beard that hyperventilation could have been responsible for the outbreak in the Royal Free Hospital, Scott stated that in her cases hyperventilation had never been observed but hypoglycaemia and abnormal glucose tolerance curves were common, as were ankle clonus, extensor plantar responses and nystagmus with a characteristic facial pallor. A careful detailed history was taken, based on a questionnaire prepared by Dr Scott and amended from time to time as further experience of the condition accrued. A diagnosis of ME was never considered unless most of the following features were present:

low-grade fever
headache
blurred vision and/or diplopia
stiff neck
vertigo with a positive Romberg test
nausea and/or vomiting
lymphadenopathy
lower costal or generalized muscular weakness
unrelieved by rest
emotional lability
insomnia and/or vivid dreams often in colour
frequency or retention of urine
varying degrees of deafness or hyperacusis

Most of the patients in this outbreak exhibited extreme tenderness in tendon sheaths and periarticular tissues, sometimes accompanied by swelling and actual fluid in the joints. In the affected limbs there was usually diminished perception to pain and touch but sometimes hyperalgesia was a prominent feature. Most patients showed emotional lability with resultant behaviour changes; some patients were morose, pessimistic and quarrelsome and wept copiously; in others the opposite was apparent in that they were overoptimistic and elated for no apparent reason. More than half the patients were discharged within a month but the more severely affected cases had repeated relapses during convalescence. Electroencephalographic and electromyographic recordings confirmed the impression of involvement of the nervous system. The involvement of joints and periosteum was regarded as quite unique but joint involvement certainly occurred among patients who are now permanently incapacitated in the aftermath of the Royal Free Hospital epidemic and in the Los Angeles outbreak (*Hart & Luck, 1936*). The authors concluded that although no viral or bacterial agent was isolated, the contagiousness of the syndrome was strongly suggestive of an infectious aetiology.

### Hospital for Sick Children, Great Ormond Street, 1970–71

An outbreak affecting the staff of the hospital between August 1970 and January 1971 was reported by Dillon and co-workers (1974). At least one hundred and forty-five cases were observed and the majority were nurses. There was the usual protean symptomatology seen in previous outbreaks and the authors stated that 'ten or eleven of the commonest symptoms were almost identical with those reported in the Royal Free Hospital outbreak in 1955'. In listing the symptoms the authors made this very striking comment:

> one symptom which does not appear in the list because it was difficult to quantify was 'rapid fatiguability reported on exercise'.

Another feature on which they commented was the 'occurrence of symptomatic relapses over a prolonged period in at least 28 patients'. Intervals between apparent recovery and relapse varied from two to six months but even during the period of recovery the patients were not restored to normal health. Some patients were free of symptoms after twelve months but in others, symptomatic relapses occurred for several years after the initial illness. The most important outcome of the laboratory investigations was the 'high incidence of anti-complementary activity in the complement-fixation antibody tests'. Of fourteen acute-phase sera, twelve (83%) were anti-complementary and of sixteen convalescent-phase sera, seven (43%) showed a similar abnormality. On immune electron microscopy, ill-defined aggregates were found in some of the sera, more particularly those shown to have anti-complementary activity.

Although no children were affected during the outbreak, Dillon and his co-workers reported that 'several children have recently been referred to the hospital with symptoms in keeping with the disease. The symptoms and signs found in these children were very similar to those recorded in the adult population in 1970.'

## An outbreak in West Kilbride, Ayrshire, 1980–83

Between January 1980 and June 1983 twenty-two patients were seen with suspected ME (*Fegan, Behan & Bell, 1983*). Of the twenty-two patients, sixteen were females aged between 8 and 53 years and six were males aged between 10 and 41 years. The disease presented as either an acute or a subacute illness. The acute symptoms consisted of vertigo, hyperacusis and tinnitus; other patients complained of chest pains on exertion, often with palpitations. Some patients developed an acute anxiety state while in a few there was reversal of sleep rhythm with early morning wakening. Patients with a subacute onset noticed increasing anxiety, depression without a cause, muscle pain and aches, coarse muscle twitchings and odd paraesthesiae. **Once the disease was established the most characteristic symptom was extreme exhaustion, particularly after exercise. The exhaustion also occurred after emotional or mental strain.**

Virological investigations showed that eighteen (82%) of the twenty-two patients had elevated neutralizing antibody titres to Coxsackie B virus. Twelve of the eighteen Coxsackie B-'positive' patients had symptoms which persisted for at least six months. The authors referred to previous studies which suggested that the higher the titre observed, the greater is the possibility of recent infection. Nine hundred and fifty normal adults in the West of Scotland had been tested for the presence of Coxsackie B neutralizing antibody; titres of 1:512 or more were found in only 4% and titres of 1:256 in 10%. In the Ayrshire series, the figures were 59% for 1:512 and above, and 55% for 1:256. It therefore seems reasonable to conclude that Coxsackie Group B viruses were responsible for the outbreak. One of the cases was a 41-year-old airline steward whose onset was precipitated followed a bicycle ride; he was at first thought to have myocardial ischaemia but further questioning elicited the fact that he had had curious feelings of panic at work with no specific provocation, increased irritability and anxiety, sleep disturbances with early morning wakening, fine 'true' vertigo, night sweats, pain in the arms and legs, and diarrhoea. His Coxsackie antibody titre was 1:1024. This type of history with precipitate onset, usually taking the form of vertigo, is by no means uncommon but it was the subsequent history that particularly aroused my interest. Several weeks later his 8-year-old daughter became unwell. Her symptoms were exhaustion with rapid fatigue on exertion. She had vague muscle pains and felt dizzy; she began to fall asleep in class and attendance at school became impossible. The Coxsackie B neutralizing antibody titre was 1:1024 and convalescence was prolonged. The remaining members of his family, namely his wife and young son, were unaffected. I have known similar instances of 'contact' cases in a family or group in which one of the contacts developed the disease while others escaped. Consequently, I had long harboured a suspicion that the triggering factor in ME is to be found in the immunological state of the patient and research is showing that this might be the case.

### Outbreak in Balfron, Stirlingshire
The outbreak in West Kilbride prompted Dr B.D. Keighley, a general practitioner in Balfron, to investigate patients in his rural practice whose protracted and atypical illnesses appeared to be similar to those seen in Ayrshire. In cooperation with Dr E.J. Bell, Top Grade Virologist at Ruchill Hospital, Glasgow, twenty patients were selected for virological studies (*Keighley & Bell, 1983*). Of the twenty patients, seventeen had suspected ME. Virological studies showed similar results to those found in West Kilbride and the results were also compared with a control group of one hundred normal adults in the west of Scotland. They arrived at a similar conclusion, namely, that the figures in their cases were significantly different from those of the normal adult population. Finally, they made this cogent observation:

If our results are considered valid and the figure of incidence in a practice comprising 2500 adults can be extrapolated to the

26

general population, then there are a large number of ill and unhappy patients in the community and it is suspected that many of these are to be found among returning attenders at medical and psychological clinics.

## Coxsackie B infection in a Scottish general practice

Prompted by the reports of the outbreaks in West Kilbride and Balfron, Calder & Warnock (1984) described thirty-eight cases of protracted illness in Helensburgh, characterized by multisystem symptomatology. They investigated eighty-one cases between 1978 and August 1983; of these, thirty-eight (47%) were found to have significantly raised antibody titres (that is 1:256 or more) to Coxsackie Group B viruses. Six other patients had borderline titres of 1:128. There were no rising antibody titres, indicating that infection was well established before the investigation. The illness bore a close resemblance to descriptions of ME which were reviewed by Behan (1980). The disease ran a fluctuating course of relapse and remission over many months and even persisted for several years. The results confirmed the results of Keighley & Bell (1983). Their increased awareness of the syndrome has led Drs Calder & Warnock to find new cases and at the time of their report they stated, 'there is no sign of a fall in incidence'. They observed that previous reports had generally dealt with epidemics rather than the sporadic or endemic pattern which their cases had followed. That observation conforms with the findings of Dr Betty Scott and myself that the disease is primarily endemic.

# 3

## The endemic form of the disease

### Synopsis

Myalgic encephalomyelitis is an **endemic** disease which is subject to periodic outbreaks of **epidemic** prevalence. Outbreaks such as those in Los Angeles, Iceland and Durban were undoubted epidemics with rapid case-to-case spread, but the outbreaks in North-West London in 1955 and Finchley in 1964 consisted of groups of sporadic cases with no history of known contact with infectious cases. It is interesting that in the recent outbreak in Helensburgh, Calder & Warnock drew attention to the same phenomenon of a sporadic or endemic pattern in their cases.

I am now in no doubt that ME is an endemic disease which is subject to periodic outbreaks of an epidemic kind. Acheson (1959) stated that, 'the first endemic case in which a diagnosis of "Iceland Disease" was made was reported by Hardtke in 1955'. Jellinek (1956) reported two such cases in Hampshire, and Galpine & Brady (1957) reported seven cases 'which arose sporadically in Coventry in the late summer of 1956'. For several years cases of this kind have been referred to me from various parts of the United Kingdom and after the outbreak in Finchley in 1964 Dr Betty Scott collaborated with me in a study of upwards of fifty patients, none of whom had been associated with an outbreak of the disease. Correspondence began to build up with doctors in the United States, Australia and New Zealand who were encountering similar problems. Many of these sufferers were doctors themselves or their wives. Indeed the number of doctors who are victims of the disease is quite out of proportion to their numbers in the population as a whole. I know of no possible explanation for this.

The patients whom Dr Scott and I saw came to us in a state of utter despair, their medical advisers finding themselves baffled by a medley of symptoms which they were unable to place into any recognizable category of disease. Without exception, these patients had been referred for consultant opinion and they were generally seen by neurologists who were equally nonplussed, having found no abnormality on physical examination and with extensive laboratory investigations failing to yield a clue. I must add, however, that in no case had any investigation of the immune system been carried out. Many of these patients were finally referred for psychiatric opinion and it is interesting that four psychiatrists to my knowledge referred patients back with a note which in essence said 'I do not know what this patient is suffering from, but the case does not come into my field'. For the most part these unfortunate people were finally rejected as hopeless neurotics and there was at least one instance of a family breaking up when five doctors assured the husband that there was nothing wrong with his wife; she is now a chronic ME sufferer with permanent physical incapacity.

Dr Scott's experience in the Finchley outbreak proved invaluable. Her very thorough study of the patients under her care at that time and their subsequent careful follow-up went a long way towards our recognition of the endemic form of the disease, as she was able to indicate features of which I had not been aware. To give one example, she pointed out that, if both sides were affected, the muscle weakness was always greater in the muscles which the patient used most in daily activities; thus, in a right-handed person, the muscles of the left arm and hand were stronger than those on the right. Dr Scott and I found that the endemic case has a well-defined and, with experience, an easily recognizable pattern, albeit one which is not taught to medical students and this may provide an explanation as to why many doctors disregard or fail to notice certain vital points.

The onset of the disease is similar to those described in the various recorded outbreaks. Thus it may be sudden and without apparent cause, as in cases where the first intimation of illness is an alarming attack of acute vertigo, but usually there is a history of infection of the upper respiratory tract or, occasionally, the gastrointestinal tract with nausea and/or vomiting. Instead of an uneventful recovery the patient is dogged by persistent and profound fatigue accompanied by a medley of symptoms such as headache, giddiness, muscle pain, cramps or twitchings, muscle tenderness and weakness, paraesthesiae, frequency of micturition, blurred vision and/or diplopia, hyperacusis (sometimes alternating with deafness or normal hearing), tinnitus and a general sense of 'feeling awful'. Some patients report the occurrence of fainting attacks relieved by a small meal or just eating a biscuit; these attacks are the result of hypoglycaemia and we are reminded of the three young women in the outbreak in Finchley who were admitted to hospital in an unconscious state, the result of acute hypoglycaemia. All cases run a low-grade pyrexia, seldom exceeding 100°F (c.38°C) and usually subsiding within a week. A very thorough examination of the central nervous system should be made and this should be accompanied by a careful estimation of muscle power, especially in the limbs and neck. A search for enlarged lymph nodes should never be omitted. If muscle power is found to be satisfactory, a re-examination should be made after exercise; a walk of half a mile is sufficient, as very few ME cases can manage more.

This phenomenon of muscle fatigability is the dominant and most persistent feature of the disease and in my opinion a diagnosis should not be made without it. Restoration of muscle power after exertion can take three to five days or even longer. It has always been my practice carefully to palpate affected muscles with the tip of the finger as tiny minute foci of exquisite tenderness can sometimes be detected; these are most likely to be found in the trapezii and gastrocnemii. I have also noted them in the abdominal recti.

In suspected cases of ME the questionnaire should include a reference to the patient's susceptibility to cold and climatic change. Practically without exception the ME patient complains of coldness of the extremities and hypersensitivity to climatic change. Impairment of the circulation is evident in the ashen-grey facial pallor which is often noted by friends or relatives some twenty minutes before the patient complains of feeling ill. In the most severe cases there may be 'crises' of acute sweating with hypothermia. I first encountered this several years ago in an ME patient who used to awaken in the night to find himself lying in a pool of water; his wife is a nurse and reports that his temperature in these episodes is 94 or 95°F (*c*.35°C). I saw him six months ago and he is still subject to these attacks. It could be attributable to damage in the region of the hypothalamus.

The third component of what I have always regarded as the 'diagnostic triad' of ME is cerebral involvement. This generally takes the form of impairment of memory and inability to concentrate. Some patients report vivid nightmares, often in colour, which they had never previously experienced. Emotional lability is a very common feature of the disease and this can prove embarrassing to patients who had prided themselves on a very stoical temperament. Two doctors have told me that they found themselves using wrong words, for example 'hot' when they meant 'cold', while the tendency to fumble with simple manoeuvres which had previously presented no difficulty is also a common occurrence in the aftermath of ME.

While some cases of ME make a complete recovery, though only after a period of many months or years, the circumstances of their individual lives may play an important part. Thus the young mother with several restless children is in an especially unfortunate position, as she cannot possibly get the rest which is essential for recovery. Absolute rest in the early stages of the disease can prove a very strong determining factor in the outcome. Relapses resulting from excessive physical and/or mental stress or after a further virus infection are an accepted feature of the disease. In most cases there is fluctuation in symptoms from one day to another or from one part of the day to another. Some never recover fully and become chronic sufferers, with permanent muscular weakness and restriction of movement due to joint involvement. A small group of patients recover completely but are subject to relapses even after a period of several years. Dr Gordon Parish, whose case I mentioned above, has gone as long as four years in perfectly sound health, yet his last relapse incapacitated him for six months and compelled him to take early retirement. A senior consultant physician who was a victim of the 1955 outbreak tells me that it was ten years before she was restored to normal health. A busy general practitioner battled on bravely for twenty-one years before she recognized that the disease was at last abating; she exhibited the typical ashen-grey facial pallor so that I could tell at a glance when she was struggling with a recrudescence of symptoms.

Another doctor in general practice begged me to obtain his retirement from NHS practice at the age of 57 years, when he knew that he was unable to do justice to his patients. I had some difficulty in persuading the DHSS that ME was a very real disease. One of the most severe cases I have encountered is the wife of a doctor in a northern industrial town; she was a prominent amateur athlete until the age of 22 when she contracted 'flu'. Since then she has battled with the muscle fatigability of ME for over forty years; during that time she has been seen by several consultant physicians who could find no cause for her symptoms and virtually pronounced her 'neurotic'; one of her daughters has developed the same condition. One of our most severely incapacitated patients was a senior technician in the Blood Transfusion Service and her chief tells me she was the author of several important papers which are regarded as 'classical' in the specialty. He now finds that he can hardly recognize her for the active person she once was. I made the diagnosis of ME in 1969 when I was asked to see her and her 12-year-old son by their doctor in Sutton. Ten years later, at the age of 22 and a student at Reading University, he was still struggling with the aftermath of the disease, which took the form of complete reversal of sleep rhythm, when sheer despair drove him to suicide by taking an overdose of nitrazepam. His mother applied for invalidity benefit and was seen by a senior neurologist who considered her to be a case of 'near-delusional self-deception' and described ME as a 'figment of the imagination both on the part of the patients who think they are suffering from it and the doctors who make the diagnosis'. The prejudice harboured against those of us who hold the view that ME is an organically determined disease defies rational explanation.

# 4

## The hypothesis of 'mass hysteria'

### Synopsis
The events leading up to the McEvedy & Beard papers in 1970 which suggested that the outbreak in the Royal Free Hospital was the result of *pure* 'mass hysteria' are described. The suggestion was made that the outbreaks in Los Angeles, Iceland and Durban and other centres were also instances of the same mechanism. Reasons are given why this hypothesis is completely untenable. Allusion is made to a paper by R.E. Kendall describing severe psychiatric disturbances following illnesses consistent with myalgic encephalomyelitis.

In the late 1960s the consultant staff of the Royal Free Hospital received a request from Drs McEvedy and Beard of the Department of Psychological Medicine at the Middlesex Hospital for permission to peruse the records of the nurses involved in the outbreak of 1955. I was one of many on the staff who saw no valid reason why this request should not be granted, as we certainly had nothing to hide. I think I am correct in saying that the only dissenting voice was that of the late Dr Helen Dimsdale, consultant neurologist; I was frankly puzzled as to the reasons for her attitude, but when I asked for an explanation she would only say, 'I think it is very possible that you will live to rue the day when you made yourself party to this decision'. No truer word was ever spoken. However, permission was granted on the understanding that the study was designed to determine a possible predisposition to psychoneurosis in the affected group. The first paper (*McEvedy & Beard, 1970a*) gave their reasons for regarding the Royal Free Hospital as an instance of 'mass hysteria'; in a second paper (*1970b*) they argued that the fourteen outbreaks reviewed by Acheson (1959) contained features which justified a similar conclusion but they agreed that 'the Los Angeles and other outbreaks associated with poliomyelitis cannot be considered such "pure" examples of mass hysteria as the Royal Free Hospital epidemic'. Drs Compston, Richardson, Dimsdale and myself (*Compston* et al., *1970*) immediately replied to this claim with a letter in which we stated that 'while a diagnosis of hysteria had been seriously considered at the time of the outbreak, the occurrence of fever in 89%, of lymphadenopathy in 79%, of ocular palsy in 43% and of facial palsy in 19% rendered it quite untenable'. In the same issue, Acheson, who had personal experience of the cases at the Middlesex Hospital in 1952, stated that they too had considered a possible diagnosis of hysteria but for similar reasons had ruled it out. Nevertheless, the McEvedy & Beard hypothesis was seized upon by the popular press (including the American *Time* magazine) as an authoritarian statement of fact from which there could be no possible appeal. Even Dr Alfred Byrne, medical correspondent of the *Sunday Times*, appeared to accept the views expressed, without question or demur. Yet neither McEvedy nor Beard had any personal experience of the disease. Their interest had been aroused as a result of an outbreak in their own hospital in 1952 (see page 16) which had been reported by Acheson (1954).

McEvedy & Beard took as the basis for their argument the fact that the epidemic of fourteen cases had occupied a fifth of a year and that, based on figures from 1950, it could be expected that two hundred and fifty nurses would report sick in that time and that thirty of them would be sufficiently ill to require admission. This was a large enough flow to provide for an epidemic of fourteen cases if all cases not immediately diagnosable as something else were regarded as 'query polio'. They therefore concluded that the 'epidemic' was an artefact due to an altered medical perception of the community and that the corollary to this view is that the syndrome which character-ized the patients after admission was due to a rising anxiety level on the part of the patients who were under threat of paralysis and a concentration of medical examination on the central nervous system. They concluded that 'the 14 patients became a homogeneous group only after admission and the symptoms then produced were due to a pre-occupation with poliomyelitis on the part of both doctors and patients'. This is a most extraordinary piece of reasoning since Acheson specifically states that 'no case of poliomyelitis or encephalo-myelitis had been nursed in the hospital in the previous month nor had any case of these diseases been notified from the adjoining boroughs'. Moreover, I have already pointed out that Case No.2 in Acheson's report (see page 17) is in itself a complete refutation of the 'hysteria' hypothesis.

I think it is only fair to say that McEvedy was probably influenced by the 'epidemic of overbreathing among schoolgirls' in Blackburn (*Moss & McEvedy, 1966*). He was further involved in two school epidemics of which the one at Portsmouth (*McEvedy, Griffith &*

*Hall, 1966*) satisfied criteria previously suggested for functional outbreaks and in which it was concluded that 'the data collected were incompatible with an organic illness'. It may well be that he was thus encouraged to bring the Royal Free Hospital and other outbreaks under similar scrutiny. Nevertheless, there can be no shred of doubt that in so doing they over-reached themselves. I have already shown that the Royal Free Hospital outbreak arose explosively from a nidus of infection which had been present in the population of North West London, that a similar nidus of infection was present in Cumbria from the beginning of the year, and that these presented in the classical form of an infectious entity with low-grade fever and generalized lymphadenopathy; to this was added the unquestionable evidence of involvement of the central nervous system with ocular and facial palsies and bulbar paralysis requiring tube-feeding. Crowley and co-workers (1957) were in no doubt that 'the course of the illness is wholly consistent with changing phases of a host–parasite relationship which are reflected in the clinical picture' and they proceeded to trace with unerring accuracy these phases:

First, during the period of invasion, the parasite left traces of its passing in the pharynx and the regional lymphatic filter. Secondly, until the sudden onset of neurological disorder after several days, the disease was often silent, except in those who displayed tenderness of muscles, glands, liver or spleen. This interval allowed time for an organism to disseminate, to pass the reticulo-endothelial defence barrier with greater or less ease in different hosts, and to multiply in the susceptible tissue before the pathogenic effect became clinically observable in the nervous system. Thirdly, the morphological changes in mature lymphocytes and altered ratio of immature to mature mononuclear cells in the blood was additional evidence of activity in the antibody forming cells of the host.

That an hysterical or functional overlay is present in many cases of ME is not in contention; indeed comment on this and the salient features of emotional lability appears in most accounts of the disease. Behan & Behan (1980) stated that had it not been for their immunological studies 'it would have been easy to concur with McEvedy and Beard that the illness is entirely a manifestation of

35

hysteria'. Against such a conclusion was the presence of generalized lymphadenopathy and of atypical lymphocytes in the peripheral blood of two patients suggestive of persistent antigenic stimulation. These findings corresponded with those of Dillon and co-workers (1974) that lymphocytes from four children with ME grew and multiplied in tissue culture, which was also a phenomenon strongly in favour of a persistent virus.

Albrecht, Oliver & Poskanzer (1964) commented that

physicians unfamiliar with the peculiar characteristics of previous epidemics . . . might easily dismiss these cases as hysteria . . . but that facile diagnosis is inadequate for reasons given by Acheson [1959] in his review of the subject as a whole . . . the mental symptoms of depression, emotional lability, impairment of memory and difficulty in concentration are consistent with organic brain disturbance and are different from the 'shallowness of affect' and 'belle indifference' of hysteria. In addition, symptoms and findings are consistent from outbreak to outbreak, in different countries, in different years, in different peoples.

In his review of the Los Angeles outbreak, Acheson (1954) quotes directly from Gilliam's (1938) original shrewd observations as follows:

the emotional upsets are difficult to interpret. They vary in degree from relatively slight displays of irritability and impatience to violent dislikes of people and things formerly liked. A common type of upset takes the form of unprovoked bouts of weeping. The emotional upsets of a few people were undoubtedly hysterical but it would be manifestly erroneous to consider as hysteria the emotional instability associated with this illness in all the cases in which it was present.

Poskanzer (1970) wrote that

the question of 'mass hysteria' had been discarded for a number of reasons, namely, cases occurring within the same household are varied in their features and course, separate illnesses appear at random intervals instead of simultaneously, epidemiologically the consistency of the course and similarity of symptoms despite the variety of people and communities that were affected make hysteria unlikely. The disease is consistent from outbreak to outbreak, in different countries, different years and different peoples and finally the mental symptoms of depression, emotional lability, impaired memory and powers of concentration are consistent with organic disease as compared with the shallowness and indifference of hysteria.

I think that McEvedy & Beard made the most damning indictment of their own hypothesis when they observed, very glibly, that in the Los Angeles and Durban outbreaks, when the medical staff were dealing with a poliomyelitis epidemic in the outside community, 'the simple explanation is surely that a bona fide polio epidemic was the initiating stress for an hysterical response by the nursing community', but they conveniently fail to record that in the Los Angeles outbreak 55% of the staff were still unfit for duty six months later and that in the Durban outbreak 'eleven patients were still disabled after three years and ten of these have been invalided out of the service while the remaining one, a senior sister, is on duty with a permanent foot-drop' (*Hill, Cheetham & Wallace, 1959*).

Subsequent events in Iceland rendered the hypothesis of 'mass hysteria' completely untenable. The spread of an extensive epidemic of Type 1 poliomyelitis in 1955 was blocked in Akureyri and two other centres where epidemic neuromyasthenia had occurred in 1948–49, and no evidence of antibody to Type 1 poliomyelitis virus was found in any of the children tested in these communities in 1956 (*Sigurdsson, Gudnadottir & Petursson, 1958*). Children without detectable antibody to any type of poliovirus were vaccinated against poliomyelitis in one of these townships, Thorshofn. A similar group of children were vaccinated against poliomyelitis in another town, Egilsstadir, in which there had been no cases of either of the two epidemic diseases. In Egilsstadir the rise in antibody titre to all three types of polio virus was poor, but in Thorshofn there was a relatively good rise to Types 2 and 3 and a negligible titre to Type 1 (*Sigurdsson, Gudnadottir & Petursson, 1958*). These results suggested that there may have been an altered immunological response to the Type 1 poliomyelitis virus in children exposed to epidemic neuromyasthenia, so that they failed to develop clinical poliomyelitis, but there was an increased response to subsequent vaccination with Type 2 and Type 3 polio virus. Parish (1974) refers to other viruses which also have an inhibiting effect on the pathological effects of poliomyelitis virus.

In 1955, Gudmundsson re-examined thirty-nine patients affected in the 1948 Akureyri epidemic and found that of those most severely affected only 25% had fully recovered and of those mildly affected only 44% had fully recovered. Moreover, 52% in the first group had residual muscular tenderness and 65% had objective neurological signs. In the second group, 50% had residual muscular tenderness and 19% had objective neurological signs (*Sigurdsson & Gudmundsson, 1956*).

Kendell (1967) described the psychiatric sequelae in two young women whose overall clinical picture was very typical of myalgic encephalomyelitis while 'both showed the almost pathognomonic electromyographic changes described by Richardson (1956)'. Both developed severe and long-lasting changes in mood and behaviour and while 'both patients had shown some evidence of neurotic predisposition beforehand', Kendell maintained that 'damage to the cerebral mechanisms underlying the control of mood and behaviour must be postulated to underlie such severe and prolonged disturbances'.

I have now given the salient features of a series of outbreaks from Los Angeles in 1934 to Scotland in 1980. The similarities in respect of mode of onset, symptomatology and prolonged aftermath with a tendency to recrudescence and relapse, with permanent incapacity in many individuals, are most striking.

All the outbreaks, together with the many sporadic ones which constitute an 'endemic' basis for the disease are bound together as a single infectious disease entity by the almost unique form of **muscle fatigability** which may in some instances result in permanent physical incapacity. I consider the McEvedy & Beard hypothesis to be totally untenable and it is a matter for regret that it was ever put forward, nor can one explain why it was accepted so readily by the profession as a whole. The records I have quoted were there to be studied at the time McEvedy & Beard published their papers and I can only hope that my account will stimulate others to check the facts for themselves. So radically did McEvedy & Beard influence medical opinion that when I have attempted to put the case for an organic explanation of the disease to younger present-day consultants I have encountered an attitude of pitying disbelief and the remark, 'Oh but that was long ago shown to have been the result of mass hysteria'. I can only say that a whole generation of unfortunate victims of the disease have been driven to despair by the failure of their doctors to recognize the validity of their symptoms. It is not surprising that six have committed suicide.

# 5

---

## Research projects

---

### Synopsis

This constitutes a brief account of the research carried out to date. Since 1978 work has been carried out in the Department of Neurology and Pathology, Glasgow, under the direction of Dr P.O. Behan, consultant neurologist, Southern General Hospital, Glasgow, together with Dr Eleanor Bell of the Enterovirus Reference Laboratory, Ruchill Hospital, Glasgow. The clinical, pathological, electrophysiological, immunological and virological abnormalities in patients with the postviral fatigue syndrome have been recorded and the findings confirm the organic nature of the disease. A study based on single-fibre electromyography has confirmed the muscle fibre is a major site of involvement.

### The Glasgow research project

At the symposium held at the Royal Society of Medicine in April 1978, Dr Peter Behan presented a paper on the subject of 'Post infectious encephalomyelitis' in which he showed that acute disseminated encephalomyelitis (ADEM) and myalgic encephalomyelitis or epidemic neuromyasthenia may share a common pathogenesis. He referred to the views of Miller, Stanton & Gibbons (1956) that ADEM usually occurs after a banal virus infection yet the disease receives little attention in textbooks of neurology, is mentioned only briefly in textbooks of medicine and is rarely considered in textbooks of psychiatry. Nevertheless it is relatively common, constituting one-third of all cases diagnosed as encephalitis (*Scott, 1967*) and is often clinically indistinguishable from multiple sclerosis. Dr Behan stressed that ADEM 'has a wide spectrum of clinical presentation' since 'it may present as a fulminating encephalitis ending fatally after a few days' or 'it can be an illness clinically indistinguishable from EME'.

Behan's initial research showed that patients with epidemic myalgic encephalomyelitis had immunological abnormalities consisting of: (1) atypical peripheral lymphocytes; (2) mild eosinophilia and anti-complementary activity; (3) increased IgM; (4) decreased or deficient IgA; (5) reduced complement factor C4 concentrations; (6) serum anti-complementary activity; and (7) a suggestion of increased titres to Coxsackie virus (in some patients specific IgM to Coxsackie virus type A9). Increased serum lactic dehydrogenase (LDH) concentrations, abnormal cerebrospinal fluid results, and abnormalities in electromyography and visual evoked-response testing represented a body of circumstantial evidence that supported the hypothesis of an organically determined disease.

This became the basis of a research project (*Behan & Behan, 1980*) in which they considered a series of forty-three outbreaks that had occurred between 1950 and 1977. They then reported their findings in a series of twelve patients who presented with the symptoms and physical signs that corresponded with those found in the various outbreaks (see Chapters 2 & 3). The symptoms included headache, pain in the neck, back and limb muscles, fatigue, exhaustion, emotional lability, irritability, poor memory, difficulty in concentration, dizziness, sore throat, diarrhoea and general malaise; physical findings included muscle tenderness, neck stiffness, pareses, lymphadenopathy, increased tendon reflexes, muscle twitchings, sensory loss, extensor plantar responses, conjunctivitis, nystagmus, cranial nerve palsies, urinary retention and respiratory failure; in brief, all the features that characterized the North West London and Royal Free Hospital outbreaks. Nevertheless, Behan & Behan stated that had it not been for the immunological studies which they carried out 'it would have been easy to concur with McEvedy and Beard that the illness is entirely a manifestation of hysteria'. But they added, 'the presence of generalised lymphadenopathy is strongly in favour of an infective process'. Moreover, the presence of atypical lymphoblasts (immunocytes) in the peripheral blood of two of the patients was suggestive of a persistent antigenic stimulation, possibly caused by a virus, and this corresponded with the findings of Dillon and co-workers (1974) who found that lymphocytes from four children grew and multiplied in tissue culture, a phenomenon strongly suggestive of a persistent virus. The presence of eosinophils in the peripheral blood of three patients suggested an allergic element in the reaction. Increased concentrations of IgM and decreased concentrations of IgA were found in half the cases. Autoantibodies were also commonly found, adding further support to the possibility of a disturbance in the immune system. The complement results together with anti-complementary activity suggested the presence of circulating immune complexes which is in line with the findings of Dillon and co-workers (1974).

Increased serum lactic dehydrogenase was found in nine of the twelve patients and this corresponded with the findings of Rundle & Ramsay (as reported in *Lyle & Chamberlain, 1978*). This is clearly indicative of muscle involvement. All routine tests on the cerebro-spinal fluid were normal but in three cases there were 'faint but definite oligoclonal bands on electrophoresis of concentrated CSF'. This finding, together with abnormal evoked visual responses, indicates involvement of the white matter of the central nervous system. It is well known that Coxsackie viruses have a predilection for cardiac and skeletal muscle and in the 1965 Coxsackie Group B5 outbreak in Europe both carditis and meningitis were found (*British Medical Journal, leading article, 1967*); Coxsackie viruses are also the aetiological agents of Bornholm disease. Behan & Behan found that two patients in their series had very high antibody titres to Coxsackie A9 virus and two had increased titres to Coxsackie B1. The husband and two sons of one of the patients developed an illness similar to ME in one of her relapses and the muscle biopsy of the husband showed the characteristic features of dermatomyositis. Behan & Behan (1977) pointed out that 'activation of the comple-ment system and the presence of circulating immune complexes' had been described by them where there was muscle damage thought to be due to a vasculopathy secondary to immune-complex deposition. They therefore suggested that in ME the pathogenesis may be that of a persistent virus with the formation of immune complexes and widespread deposition of antigen–antibody aggregates in the blood vessels, the central nervous system and muscle.

Behan, Behan & Bell (1985) reported a further study of fifty patients, eighteen males and thirty-two females, ranging in age from 17 to 55 years. They included five medical practitioners, eight nurses, the wives of four doctors, two medical social workers, one medical student and one hospital laboratory technician. The duration of the illness ranged from three months to twenty-two years. Cases were termed 'acute' when seen within the first six months. All patients gave a history of a viral-like illness; in three the onset was associated with varicella and in two with rubella. **All fifty had gross fatigue made worse by exercise.** Most of them also complained of depression, difficulty in concentration, varying degrees of tinnitus and a feeling of disturbed equilibrium, as well as hot and cold flushes. The illness was severe and had a disastrous effect on their lives. Four of the five medical practitioners and all eight nurses were unable to continue work. The illness became chronic in thirty-seven and ran a remitting course in thirteen.

Lymphocyte function was abnormal in the group as a whole. In thirty-five of the fifty patients it was highly abnormal; six of the thirty-five with severe lymphocyte dysfunction were examined serially and they showed the same changes for up to two years. Significant changes were found in patients with both acute and chronic postviral fatigue syndrome. All eleven patients in the acute group showed a reduction in the number of suppressor/cytotoxic T lymphocytes. Among the patients which chronic illness it was the helper/inducer T lymphocytes which were significantly reduced. Five patients were examined at intervals over periods up to two years and the decrease in helper cells was found to persist. Seventy per cent had impaired T-cell function as estimated by lymphocyte protein synthesis and this was detectable in patients for up to two years.

High titres of serum autoantibodies were found to smooth muscle in eighteen patients, to thyroglobulin in thirteen, to nuclear constituents in six and to gastric parietal cells in four.

Tests for antibodies to viruses other than Coxsackie were negative. Thirty-five of the fifty patients had antibody titres of 1:512 or greater to Coxsackie Group B viruses while in six of them specific IgM antibodies were detected.

No muscle weakness was found in any of the patients until they were exercised by squeezing the rubber ball of an ergometer for one minute or by going up forty steps; the weakness lasted for up to three hours. Muscle biopsies were abnormal in all twenty patients examined; these showed widely scattered necrotic muscle fibres in fifteen but there was no inflammatory infiltrate associated with the necrosis. Histochemical stains showed moderately increased size and numbers of type II fibres, which are concerned with inaugurating muscle movement and, by nature, fatigue rapidly in all biopsy samples. Using electron microscopy, mitochondria were seen to be conspicuously increased at the periphery of the fibres and occasional tubular inclusions were present.

The authors consider that the results of their investigation suggest that 'the syndrome is due to the interaction of viral infection and immunological processes which produce damage to intracellular enzymes and result in abnormal muscle metabolism especially on exercise'.

### Nuclear magnetic resonance
Encouraged by the report of a case of mitochondrial myopathy diagnosed by the comparatively new technique of phosphorus

nuclear magnetic resonance (P-NMR) at the Medical Research Unit at the Radcliffe Infirmary in Oxford (*Gadian* et al., *1981*), Dr Scott and I referred a young doctor whom we had been asked to see by my colleague Dr R.T.D. Emond at Coppett's Wood Hospital. He had a history of chicken pox complicated by encephalomyelitis four years previously, followed by increasing difficulty in carrying on with his practice. He told us that if he took his dog for a 2–3 mile walk he was completely exhausted for the next twenty-four hours. While it is very unusual for a patient with ME to be able to walk 2 or 3 miles, this man had been exceptionally fit in his university days when he was an enthusiastic mountaineer. During exercise in the P-NMR test he showed abnormally early intracellular acidosis of muscle. Since intracellular acidosis may be associated with muscle fatigue the patient's symptoms could have been the result of early and excessive production of lactic acid. This case was reported in full detail in the *Lancet* (*Arnold* et al., *1984*) and the authors concluded that the fatigue was more likely to have been the result of excessive glycolytic activity; this hypothesis was supported by the increased number of type II muscle fibres present.

We naturally regarded this P-NMR test as a possible specific test for ME but three established cases referred for testing proved negative. Professor G.K. Radda has recently reported that he and his group have examined over forty cases of postviral fatigue syndrome. In a private communication he informs me that P-NMR does not give consistently positive results in these cases. Exercise-induced excessive intracellular acidosis observed in the muscles of some of these patients is also observed in patients with a different history. It would therefore be unwise to give an opinion as to the value of NMR as a test for ME.

Possibly the most fundamental advance in our understanding of muscle pathology was the histological study of Byrne and his co-workers in 1985 when they reported non-specific type II-fibre atrophy in two patients with persistent neuralgia after an ill-defined systemic illness, marked fluctuations in the severity of the symptoms and normal neuromuscular examination with the exception of variable muscle tenderness. They also reported that mitochondrial respiration, assayed polarographically in intact organelles *in vitro*, revealed a mild depression of stage 3 respiration rates with site I and site II substrates. The results suggest that some patients with chronic myalgia may have a partial deficiency in oxidative phosphorylation. In the management of such cases the authors stress the importance of recognizing the possibility of an organic basis for the illness and of differentiating muscle pain of psychogenic origin.

## Muscle damage associated with viral infections

It is interesting to note that as far back as 1976 a number of papers were published showing subtle but definite changes in patients with acute viral and mycoplasma infections and similar changes in patients who had been admitted to psychiatric units for bizarre psychotic illnesses. Astrom, Friman & Pilstrom (1976) showed the effects of viral and mycoplasma infection on ultrastructure and enzyme activities in human skeletal muscle. Thus, thirteen men aged 20 to 42 with acute viral and mycoplasma infections were studied and compared with eight healthy men aged 22–29 years confined to bed for similar periods of time. The activities of four enzymes were measured; these were lower in the thirteen infected men than in the healthy controls in whom only one enzyme showed decreased activity and this was restored immediately on return to normal living. In the acute viral and mycoplasma infectious cases ultrastructural changes within the muscle were also found. Crayton & Meltzer (1976) reported structural alteration of the motor endplate in psychotic patients in whom they had noted increased muscle tone which decreased as the psychotic episode remitted. Their suspicion that the neuromuscular system was involved in the psychotic process was confirmed by abnormal elevation of serum creatine phosphokinase (CPK) levels. Exploration of the structure and physiology of muscle by biopsy was abnormal in nine of twenty-four cases tested and eight of these had increased CPK activity. In addition to the nine with abnormalities of muscle fibre, ten out of twenty-two psychotic patients had areas of Z-band disruption, indicating early pathology of the muscle fibre. They noted a strong tendency for patients with abnormal CPK values to have abnormal values for motor neuron excitability. However, Ramsay & Rundle (1979) noted no rise in CPK levels, though serum myoglobin and other enzyme levels were raised (see page 7 ).

Disturbed neuromuscular transmission in viral infections was first described by Friman, Schiller & Schwartz (1977). Fourteen subjects with influenza or ECHO virus infection, all suffering from myalgia, and nine subjects with mumps, though without myalgia, were investigated by single-fibre electromyography both in the acute phase and during convalescence. Both groups showed abnormal transmission characteristics in the acute phase but two weeks after the acute infection the percentage with disturbed neuromuscular transmission had decreased significantly in the group with myalgia while in the non-myalgic group it remained at the same level. On both occasions and in both groups the percentages were substantially greater than those recorded in healthy individuals.

A very important contribution to our understanding of muscle damage in the postviral fatigue syndrome was made by Goran Jamal and Stig Hansen working in the Glasgow University Department of Neurology. In 1985 they reported the results of single-fibre electromyography in forty patients with ME. A concentric needle electromyography (CNEMG) was performed on several muscles in each patient to exclude evidence of neuropathy or myopathy and these proved normal in all cases. Repetitive stimulation of the right ulnar nerve was also performed to exclude a gross neuromuscular transmission defect. Single-fibre electromyography was carried out on the right extensor digitorum communis muscle and recordings were made from all the patients and the 'jitter value' estimated. Grouping phenomena similar to that described by Richardson (1956) were seen in fourteen patients and in ten patients there was a reduced interference pattern without grouping. The findings of Friman, Schiller & Schwartz (1977) were fully confirmed. Despite marked increase in 'jitter values', absence of 'impulse blocking' (which usually occurs at jitter values exceeding $80-100\mu s$ in cases of neuromuscular transmission defect) made the neuromuscular junction an unlikely site of involvement. The authors concluded that it was reasonable to assume that the site of involvement was muscle fibre membrane conduction and their finding of 'few very low jitter values' was consistent with the presence of scattered muscle fibre necrosis in muscle biopsy. They claimed to have shown 'clear electrophysiological evidence of an abnormality in the peripheral part of the motor unit in patients with postviral fatigue syndrome'.

There are clearly several mechanisms by which viruses can cause muscle damage. The first is that postulated by Professor Radda, namely, excessive glycolysis. A second possible mechanism is interference with enzyme activity. On the occasion of the 5th International Congress on Neuromuscular Disease in Marseilles in 1982, Aquaronn, Cremieux & Pellissier described adenylate deaminase deficiency following virus infections. This had also been described by Shumate and co-workers (1979), who showed a marked deficiency of adenylate deaminase in six cases with varying forms of muscular weakness (two of which followed an influenzal illness). No abnormality was found on examination of the central nervous system, CPK levels were consistently normal and muscle biopsy revealed normal histochemistry with the exception of the absence of myoadenylate deaminase.

It is clear, therefore, that the mode of action of viruses on the muscle cell is extremely complex and no single line of research can provide an adequate explanation. Southern & Oldstone (1986) discussed the medical consequences of persistent viral infection. They forecast that a tremendous expansion of knowledge related to the molecular mechanisms of virus disease is expected and that in addition to molecular biology, advances in genetics, immunology and protein chemistry will also play a part. Basic questions such as how viruses infect cells, why they are liable to persist, how they evade immune surveillance and maintain a persistent state, and what underlies the ability of viruses to injure cells and tissues thereby producing disease, await answers. Once inside a cell viruses can cause destruction in multiple ways: they may block or divert enzymes necessary for cellular metabolism or replication; they may disrupt the membranes of intracellular structures and cause lethal digestive enzymes to be released; they may disrupt the cell's plasma membrane and alter its permeability sufficiently to lead to its destruction. Viral proteins inserted into the cell membrane can alter its function and integrity.

The future of medical virology will probably relate to **persistent virus infections** and in this group are included many of the herpes group of viruses which may not always kill the host cell in which they replicate, may not provoke an immune response or may not generate immune responses that are effective in clearing the virus. Southern & Oldstone also discussed both how persistent infections become established and the new concept that some viruses can cause disease not by destroying the cells that they infect but by altering the specialized function of the infected cell. They consider that such disorders involve primarily the immune, nervous and endocrine systems. All these systems, particularly the first two, are vitally involved in the pathogenesis of ME.

# 6

# Discussion

## Synopsis

I have attempted to show that the disease we know as myalgic encephalo-myelitis and which has been known in America as epidemic neuro-myasthenia is endemic, with periodic outbreaks of epidemic prevalence. The clinical findings show a very strong similarity in both the endemic and epidemic forms of the disease and are consistent with the classical form of an infectious disease process. I have discussed a possible explanation for failure to isolate the aetiological agent in the earlier outbreaks and it would seem likely that any virus may 'trigger' the disease if the immunological state of the patient is defective. The hypothesis of 'mass hysteria' is shown to be untenable. The reports in three separate papers of 'prolonged and atypical illnesses' following infection with Epstein–Barr virus in the United States show them to be virtually indistinguishable from ME.

The chronic mononucleosis syndrome is described. Evidence for a permanent viral carrier state is discussed. Allusion is made to the claim that SMON virus could be an aetiological agent of ME.

In the writing of this thesis I have had a two-fold objective. In the first place I have attempted to show that the condition we have called myalgic encephalomyelitis and which the Americans know as epidemic neuromyasthenia is basically endemic but subject to periodic outbreaks which may be justifiably designated 'epidemics' when they occur in closed communities such as hospitals or colleges where there is rapid case-to-case spread with heightened virulence of the organism; in the outbreaks in North West London and Finchley (see pp 5, 23) there were a number of sporadic cases with no history of known contact with a source of infection. The striking similarity of such outbreaks was stressed by Henderson & Shelokov (1959) and by Acheson (1959). But the importance of the clinical finding of **muscle fatigability** has not yet been stressed sufficiently. It features in every account of the disease and Behan, Behan & Bell (1985) summed it up in the statement 'all 50 patients had the same primary symptom, that of gross fatigue made worse by exercise'. Its unique nature lies in the fact that there is a prolonged delay, up to three to five days or even longer, before the restoration of muscle power after exercise is complete. In many cases this phenomenon becomes chronic. Whether occurring in endemic or epidemic form, this is the feature which binds the disease into one single clinical entity. The diagnostic difficulties presented by cases with paresis can be solved by re-examination after exercise and close interrogation regarding the effects of cold and climatic change, sweating, hypothermia, impairment of memory and powers of concentration, alteration in dream pattern and intensity, bladder disturbances and variability in hearing. While cases without paresis may resolve uneventfully within a few months, they too are subject to relapse and recrudescence in which the initial symptoms are intensified, just as severely as the case with paresis. This then constitutes the postviral fatigue syndrome, to use the recently coined term, and without it a diagnosis of ME is never justified. In short, the possibility of relapse is inherent in all cases of ME and this would seem to be precipitated by excessive physical and/or mental stress or by a further virus infection. In some cases, however, there is a definite 'periodicity' in relapses, which may occur when physical and mental stress has not been a factor, though further virus infection may be a 'trigger' for relapse. The question has arisen as to whether ME is the result of a persistent virus infection or an immunoregulatory disorder. It is not possible that both these mechanisms may play a part in causing relapse and, in so many cases, permanent disability?

There is undoubtedly an extraordinary relationship between the aetiological factor in ME and infection with poliomyelitis virus. The outbreaks in Los Angeles, Iceland, Adelaide, Coventry and Durban corresponded with epidemics of poliomyelitis. In Los Angeles the outbreak was at first considered to be 'abortive poliomyelitis', but virological and serological studies showed no evidence of poliomyelitis and the cerebrospinal fluid in all cases was normal. Finally, the clinical picture showed no evidence of wasting of muscle and wherever electromyographic studies were carried out there was no evidence of damage to the anterior horn cells in the spinal cord, thus eliminating the possibility of even an 'abortive' form of poliomyelitis. Yet, whatever the aetiological factor in ME it had a definite inhibitory effect on the pathological effects of poliomyelitis infection. This was clearly illustrated when an epidemic of Type 1 poliomyelitis in Iceland in 1955 spread around the coast but failed to become established in the four centres where epidemic neuromyasthenia had occurred in 1948. Indeed, this inhibitory effect was also apparent in Iceland in 1948 since the first three cases in Akureyri were considered to be 'classical poliomyelitis' but were thereafter supplanted by cases of epidemic neuromyasthenia. The same extraordinary inhibitory effect was seen in the Middlesex Hospital in 1952, when one of the nurses was found to have poliomyelitis virus Type 3 in her faeces, but this failed to produce any pathogenic effects, nor did the patient develop any antibody to the virus. There was also an extraordinary response to poliomyelitis vaccination reported by Sigurdsson, Gudnadottir & Petursson (1958), who showed that children in epidemic neuromyasthenia areas responded to poliomyelitis vaccination with higher antibody titres than in other areas not affected by the poliomyelitis epidemic, suggesting that these children had already been exposed to an agent immunologically similar to the poliomyelitis virus.

The nature of the aetiological agent in these earlier epidemics remains a matter of conjecture, but I think it worth referring to Parish (1974). Apparently the first indication that the classical neuropathology of anterior poliomyelitis can be modified was reported by Pappenheimer and his co-workers (1951) in a routine attempt to isolate poliomyelitis virus from a child with a typical clinical history and signs of poliomyelitis. The child's faeces contained an agent which was transmitted to monkeys, producing inflammatory and degenerative changes on the surfaces of nerve roots, especially in the lumbar and sacral regions. **The anterior horn cells were free from damage.** Parish also refers to a new clinical entity which appeared in Japan ten years previously and was thought to have features in common with outbreaks of epidemic neuromyasthenia in other parts of the world. The illness was named subacute myelo-optic neuropathy (SMON) and the virus inhibited the growth of poliomyelitis virus markedly; it was also shown to produce a disease in mice similar to human SMON. A delayed antibody response seems to result in the establishment of a subacute persistent infection producing exacerbations and remissions of the disease. Some of the nurses looking after patients with SMON had antibody to the virus, indicating that subclinical infection can occur. The properties of the SMON virus would explain many of the features of epidemic neuromyasthenia. It resembles a DNA virus of subgroup A of the herpes virus group. If SMON or similar viruses were responsible for the earlier outbreaks of ME, then it is not remarkable that virus investigations proved negative, since these viruses were not identified until 1971 (*Inoue, Nishibe & Kimura, 1971*) and they are difficult to culture.

My second objective has been to expose the McEvedy & Beard

hypothesis as completely untenable. I consider that the evidence I have provided of the frequency of relapse and chronic morbidity achieves this. Their selection of the Royal Free Hospital epidemic as an instance of ' "pure" mass hysteria' betrays an abysmal ignorance of the infectious process. As Crowley and her co-workers (1957) indicated, the progress of an infectious agent through the faeces and pharynx with the involvement of enlarged glands in all regions, the silent interval allowing time for the organism to pass the reticulo-endothelial barrier, varying in different hosts, and the ultimate lodgement in the central nervous system are clearly portrayed and this is the classical mode of presentation of a generalized infectious process. I have already alluded to Case 2 in Acheson's report on the outbreak in the Middlesex Hospital in 1952 (see page 17), in which there is clear evidence of permanent damage in the spinal cord twelve months after recovery from the infection. Finally, inhibition of the pathological effects of poliomyelitis virus infection during the epidemic of 1955 in four centres where ME had prevailed in 1948 could not by any stretch of the imagination be accounted for by 'mass hysteria'. Nor do I consider that 'mass hysteria' could account for the prolonged illness persisting for three years and compelling the retirement of ten nurses from the profession in the Durban outbreak.

Our reports on the outbreaks in North West London and the Royal Free Hospital received very favourable editorial comment. The *Lancet* (1956) referred to our report on the first eight cases in North West London as 'A New Clinical Entity?' and the subject was very fully reviewed with reference to all similar outbreaks reported up to that time. The subject was further reviewed when the *Lancet* published my report on thirty-four cases in 1957. The *British Medical Journal* gave similar prominence to the report of the physicians of the Royal Free Hospital in 1957 and a further leading article appeared in June 1978, commenting on the symposium held at the Royal Society of Medicine earlier that year.

It is quite understandable that many may consider it is premature to talk of a well-defined clinical entity of infectious origin, when evidence of a specific aetiological agent is singularly lacking, but improved methods of virus culture may fill that gap and the importance of modern techniques in virus culture is illustrated by Dr P.O. Behan's decision to select Coxsackie Group B virus as a possible aetiological agent and Dr Bell's success in identifying that organism as the causal agent of the outbreaks in West Kilbride, Balfron and Helensburgh. These authors also reported that in three

51

of their cases the onset was associated with chicken pox and in two with rubella.

Lyle (1959) described an outbreak of infectious disease in Newton-le-Willows in Lancashire which in both its acute phase and its aftermath bore a close resemblance to the outbreaks described above. ECHO 9 virus was isolated from the stools of four patients and a rising titre of neutralizing antibody to the virus was found in six. Innes (1970) described four cases of 'encephalomyelitis resembling benign myalgic encephalomyelitis'. Coxsackie B2 and ECHO 3 viruses were isolated from the cerebrospinal fluid in two cases and raised neutralizing antibody titres to Coxsackie B2 and B5 viruses were found in two cases. These points lend credence to my long-held view that it is not so much the aetiological agents, as the immuno-logical state of the patient, which determines the development of the disease. This was suggested to me several years ago, when two friends on holiday contracted the same respiratory virus infection: one recovered uneventfully, the other (a doctor) developed ME and has become a chronic sufferer.

The most important development in the unfolding of this 'saga' and one which will surely bring to an end the prejudice which has prevailed for so long against any attempt to show this disease as an organically determined entity, is the demonstration that another virus may give rise to 'prolonged and atypical illnesses' which are so similar to ME as to be indistinguishable from it. This is the Epstein–Barr virus, identified in 1964 from tissue in cases of Burkitt's lymphoma, a malignant disease found in young African women in Uganda. Epstein–Barr (EB) virus is ubiquitous and is the aetiological agent of infectious mononucleosis. It is worth recalling that during the early stage of the outbreak in the Royal Free Hospital, a diagnosis of glandular fever was considered but, with the Paul–Bunnell test proving consistently negative, the idea was finally discarded. Nevertheless the leader writer in the *British Medical Journal* of July 30, 1955, pointed out that infectious mononucleosis is a very puzzling disease and might well comprise a group of allied diseases. Thus most cases occur sporadically and are of low infectivity, and it is unusual for more than one case to occur in a family or in a hospital ward. These cases almost invariably give a true positive Paul–Bunnell test, with its characteristic absorption tests. Yet, even when severe with acute exudative tonsillitis, the infectivity remains low and this contrasts with the epidemic type in which most cases are mild and often symptomless, except for posterior cervical gland involvement. These contrasts suggest a difference in aetiology between sporadic and epidemic cases. Hoagland (1955), from a study of the sporadic disease in college students, noted its rare occurrence in room-mates and also a double peak of incidence in February and August, some five or six weeks after the end of term. In several cases he found that symptoms began thirty-three to forty-nine days after an incident of intimate kissing. He suggests that the virus may be destroyed or inhibited by dilution with saline or separation from the body, thus accounting for the failure of transmission experiments, but that it may be transmitted by intimate oral contact or by indirect transfer of saliva, as by drinking from the same bottle. His observations suggest a much longer incubation period than the usually accepted one of five to fourteen days. I can find no evidence that this work by Hoagland has ever been corroborated, but the leader writer was in no doubt that infectious mononucleosis is much more prevalent than is generally accepted and that while the course of the acute disease is rarely longer than ten to fifteen days, it may be followed by a period of weakness for some weeks or even months. My own experience in the care of students with the disease fully confirms that observation.

The leader writer in the *Lancet* of May 4, 1985, reviewed three papers which suggested that EB virus is probably responsible for unusually severe, protracted and recurrent illnesses among patients suffering from infectious mononucleosis. Tobi and co-workers (1982) produced serological evidence of persistent EB virus infection in seven patients with a 'prolonged and atypical illness' who were followed up for one year. Sera taken during that time showed significantly increased titres of IgM antibodies against the viral capsid antigen (VCA) of EB virus. Only one of these patients presented with symptoms of classical infectious mononucleosis, but nevertheless the authors considered that the illness might have been associated with an aberrant immune response and that reactivation of the EB virus, rather than a primary infection, was the underlying aetiological factor. Jones and co-workers (1985) reported that forty-four patients, including twenty-six adults and eighteen children under 15 years of age were referred for recurrent or unexplained illnesses. Symptoms included pharyngitis, fatigue, depression, dys-logia and myalgia. Thirty-nine patients had antibody to EB virus and the levels were compatible with active infection for one year. Straus, Tosato & Armstrong (1985) evaluated twenty-three patients with persistent illness and fatigue after infectious mononucleosis and found higher titres of IgG anti-VCA and antibodies to restricted components of early antigen (EACR) than in age- and sex-matched seropositive controls. Other abnormalities included circulating immune complexes and increased *in vitro* cell-mediated suppression of immunoglobulin synthesis.

I find it essential to draw attention to the considerable literature which is building up on the 'chronic mononucleosis syndrome'. Hamblin and co-workers (1983) investigated a group of patients suffering from chronic ill health after an attack of acute infectious mononucleosis and discovered a disorder of T-cell regulation. The staining pattern associated with T suppressor cells was found in a greater proportion than in normal subjects while the reverse was true for T helper cells. These patients were unwell for at least a year but most made a complete recovery and this was associated with a return to normal of the lymphocyte subsets.

The absence in the medical literature of diagnostic criteria of a chronic mononucleosis syndrome prompted Dubois and co-workers (1984) to publish data on fourteen patients who presented with the abnormal serology of reactivated EB virus infection, namely elevated IgG anti-VCA, negative IgM anti-VCA, positive anti-EA and positive EBNA (Epstein–Barr nuclear antigen) antibody titres. The absence of IgM anti-VCA and the presence of anti-EBNA antibodies indicated that these patients did not have a primary infection of pronounced T-cell deficiency, while other findings in acute infectious mononucleosis, namely lymphadenopathy, pharyngitis, high fever, abnormal liver function, splenomegaly, high-titre heterophil antibody or IgA anti-VCA titres, were absent.* The authors concluded that the chronic mononucleosis syndrome is far more common than was previously recognized but agreed that further clinical epidemiological and immunological studies were required to define the syndrome.

Borysiewicz and co-workers (1986) reported that in a number of patients recovery from infectious mononucleosis following primary infection with EB virus was complicated by the persistence of symptoms for months or years. Normal recovery from infectious

---

*VCA: viral capsid antigen
EA(D): diffuse components of early antigen
EA(R): restricted components of early antigen
EBNA: Epstein–Barr nuclear antigen
Heterophil antibody forms the basis of the Paul–Bunnell diagnostic test for acute infectious mononucleosis.

mononucleosis is associated with the development of EB virus-specific antibodies and memory cytotoxic T cells which are present in the peripheral blood of normal seropositive individuals. They studied four patients who had persistent symptoms for more than two years after infectious mononucleosis. All four patients had normal imunoglobulin concentrations, T- and B-cell numbers, T-cell proliferative responses and natural killer cell activity. However, three of the four had reduced or absent antibodies to EBNA, although other EB virus-specific antibody titres were normal. All four had reduced EB virus-specific cytotoxic T-cell activity as measured by the EB virus regression assay. These studies indicate that the syndrome of persistent symptoms following EB virus mononucleosis may be associated with a defect in EB virus-specific immunity and so suggest a possible immunological basis for the syndrome.

After a very extensive survey of chronic mononucleosis, Tobi & Morag (1984) regard Epstein–Barr virus as a common archetype of human latent viral infections and they ascribe this to its infection of B lymphocytes resulting in a permanent viral carrier state:

These genome-carrying cells may give rise to continuous EBV-containing lymphoblastoid cell lines in 'in vitro' cultures established from the peripheral blood and lymph node lympho-cytes of sero-positive individuals. Given the high incidence of exposed individuals (eighty percent by late adolescence) the recognised tendency of herpes viruses to reactivation, the persistent carrier state and the predisposition of atypical infections, it might be expected that recurrent or prolonged atypical infections would be commonly reported.

Very strong support for these views is now forthcoming. Bowles and co-workers (1986) described the detection of Coxsackie B virus-specific RNA sequences in myocardial biopsy samples from patients with myocarditis and dilated cardiomyopathy. Whereas the connection between Coxsackie Group B viruses and myocarditis is widely recognized, no direct link between virus replication and damage to the myocardium has been previously established. Endo-myocardial biopsy is apparently a safe procedure and the authors have shown that a Coxsackie Group B virus-specific DNA hybridization probe can detect virus nucleic acid sequences in a large proportion of patients diagnosed as having active or healed myocarditis or congestive cardiomyopathy. The frequency of detection (53%) shows that involvement of Coxsackie B viruses in cardiac disease is clinically important. Certain specimens positive for the presence of Coxsackie B virus obtained by late biopsy of healed myocarditis suggests that virus persists after the acute phase of the disease and disposes to the development of cardiomyopathy. Detection at the late stage of the disease implies continuing virus replication. Tilzey, Signy & Banatvala (1986) reported two patients with recurrent pericarditis who had Coxsackie-specific IgM responses for at least six years in one case and twenty months in the other. This suggests continuous antigenic stimulus and that consideration should be given to the role of this group of viruses in inducing persistent infection.

Thus we see that both Epstein-Barr and Coxsackie Group B viruses are potential aetiological factors in the postviral fatigue syndrome and in both there is evidence of a persistent carrier state.

I have referred above to SMON virus. This virus was first isolated from the cerebrospinal fluids of patients with subacute myelo-optic neuropathy (SMON) by Inoue and co-workers (1971) who later showed a serological relationship between the virus and avian infectious laryngotracheitis (*Inoue & Nishibe, 1973*). This virus is a member of the herpes group of viruses and the possibility that it could have been responsible for many of the earlier outbreaks of ME should not be dismissed lightly. The fact that it can modify the effects of poliomyelitis virus is of particular importance. Indeed, before Inoue had identified SMON virus, Okuda and his colleagues (1965) were able to isolate from a Japanese outbreak of epidemic neuromyasthenia a virus which inhibited the growth of poliomyelitis virus. This effect was neutralized by serum from one of the patients. Melnick and his colleagues in America have published several papers on a transmissable agent which they call IM virus and which is antigenically related to the Japanese SMON virus. They have isolated IM virus from cerebrospinal fluids in patients suffering from multiple sclerosis and other chronic disorders of the central nervous system (*Melnick* et al., *1984*).

The leader writer in the *Lancet* (1985) stated that 'although the observations made by Straus and his co-workers do not prove that EB virus causes chronic ill-health the evidence seems very strong' and added 'whatever the underlying mechanism – whether a continuing infection or an immuno-regulatory disorder, patients may be much helped by the knowledge that their persistent vague complaints could have an organic basis'. This is precisely what we have been striving to accomplish for the unfortunate victims of these unexplained illnesses over nearly thirty years. Jane E. Brady, writing in the *New York Times* of June 12, 1985, told the story of the unexplained illness which may follow infection with EB virus and referred to the papers by Jones and co-workers (1985) and Straus and co-workers (1985). But the story she told of the misery endured by sufferers whose illnesses elude medical diagnosis was identical with the story of the many victims of myalgic encephalomyelitis over a period that goes back at least fifty years. The post Epstein–Barr virus infection is 'spot-on' ME. Research in the United Kingdom and in the United States has now confirmed a link between both Epstein–Barr and Coxsackie Group B viruses and the postviral fatigue syndrome.

So we have virtually reached the end of 'The saga of Royal Free disease' and the victims of ME should no longer have to dread the verdict of, 'All your tests are normal. Therefore nothing is wrong with you'.

## Treatment

The basic essential in treatment is correct diagnosis. That is a truism which might be said to apply to all human ailments but I have never seen it so vividly illustrated as in victims of ME. Many of these sufferers have been referred over a span of several months or years to various authorities without being able to obtain a definite diagnosis. Most have been labelled 'depression' and, finally, 'neurosis'. When they are told that their illness has a name and is not 'all in the mind' and they receive a measure of reassurance regarding their future, one can see the mantle of depression fall from their shoulders as fresh hope dawns. Indeed the 'depression' may not be real but the result of utter despair, although true depression does occur in some cases. One can hold out no specific 'cure' for the illness but advice should immediately be given that they adapt their lives to a quieter tempo and take adequate periods of complete rest after physical exertion. It is at this point that the Patient's Association comes into the picture to provide a therapy the value of which is beyond computation. It can refer members to others in their vicinity who are in a similar plight. This has led to the formation of Groups which meet at regular intervals to exchange experiences and to discuss information supplied by the Association. This leads to a restoration of inner spiritual resources which alone can provide the staying power to face what may prove to be a long period of physical incapacity. Many doctors and their wives suffer from ME and I have found that their period of recovery varies from ten to twenty years. Some have to face permanent incapacity and Dr Behan and I have been instrumental in obtaining early retirement for a few doctors who found that they were not in a fit state to carry on general practice. One of them has described his experience of ME in articles to the press and also spoke on the radio programme 'Medicine Now'.

Two methods of therapy have been tried: the administration of immunoglobulins; and the anti-viral agent inosine pranobex (Immunovir). I have no personal experience of these but a close analysis of the former will be undertaken shortly under the direction of Professor James Mowbray at St Mary's Hospital. Allergies are a frequent complicating factor in patients with immunodeficiency and their treatment should be managed by physicians who have specialized in that field.

# References

Acheson, E.D. (1954) Encephalomyelitis associated with poliomyelitis virus. *Lancet*, **2**, 1044–1048

Acheson, E.D. (1959) The clinical syndrome variously called Benign Myalgic Encephalomyelitis, Iceland Disease and Epidemic Neuromyasthenia. *American Journal of Medicine*, **26**, 569–595

Albrecht, R.M., Oliver, V.L. & Poskanzer, D.C. (1964) Epidemic Neuromyasthenia. Outbreak in a convent in New York State. *Journal of the American Medical Association*, **187**, 904–907

Aquaronn, R., Mante, S., Cremieux, G. & Pellissier, J.F. (1982) Myoadenylate deaminase deficiency. 5th International Congress on Neuromuscular Diseases, Marseilles. Abstract TU17.

Arnold, D.I., Bore, P.J., Radda, G.K., Styles, P. & Taylor, D.J. (1984) Excessive intracellular acidosis of skeletal muscle on exercise in a patient with a post viral fatigue syndrome. *Lancet*, **1**, 1367–1369

Astrom, E., Friman, G. & Pilstrom, L. (1976) Effects of viral and mycoplasma infection on ultrastructure and enzyme activities in human skeletal muscle. *Acta pathologica et microbiologica Scandinavica, Section A*, **84**, 113–122

Behan, P.O. (1978) Post-infectious encephalomyelitis: some aetiological mechanisms. *Postgraduate Medical Journal*, **54**, 755–759

Behan, P.O. (1980) Epidemic Encephalomyelitis. *Practitioner*, **224**, 805–807

Behan, P.O. & Behan, W.M.H. (1980) Epidemic myalgic encephalomyelitis. In *Clinical Neuroepidemiology*, pp.374–383. London: Pitman Medical

Behan, P.O., Behan, W.M.H. & Bell, E.J. (1985) The postviral fatigue syndrome: an analysis of the findings in 50 cases. *Journal of Infection*, **10**, 211–222

Behan, W.M.H. & Behan, P.O. (1977) Complement abnormalities in polymyositis. *Journal of Neurological Science*, **34**, 241–246

Borysiewicz, I.K., Haworth, S.J., Cohen, J., Mundin, J., Rickinson, A. & Sissona, J.G.D. (1986) Epstein-Barr virus-specific immune defects in patients with persistent symptoms following infectious mononucleosis. *Quarterly Journal of Medicine*, **58**, 111–121

Bowles, N.E., Olsen, E.G.L., Richardson, P.J. & Archard, L.C. (1986) Detection of Coxsackie B virus-specific RNA sequences in myocardial biopsy samples from patients with myocarditis and dilated cardiomyopathy. *Lancet*, **1**, 1120

Byrne, E., Trounce, I. & Dennett, X. (1985) Chronic Relapsing Myalgia. *Australian and New Zealand Journal of Medicine*, **15**, 305–308

Calder, B.D. & Warnock, P.J. (1984) Coxsackie B infection in a Scottish general practice. *Journal of the Royal College of General Practitioners*, **34**, 15–19

Compston, N.D. (1978) An outbreak of encephalomyelitis in the Royal Free Hospital Group in 1955. *Postgraduate Medical Journal*, **54**, 722–724

Compston, N.D., Dimsdale, H.E., Ramsay, A.M. & Richardson, A.T. (1970) Epidemic malaise. *British Medical Journal*, **1**, 170–171

Crayton, J.W. & Meltzer, H.Y. (1976) Motor endplate alterations in schizophrenic patients. *Nature*, **264**, 658–659

Crowley, N., Nelson, M. & Stovin, S. (1957) Epidemiological aspects of an outbreak of encephalomyelitis at the Royal Free Hospital in the summer of 1955. *Journal of Hygiene (Cambridge)*, **55**, 102–122

Daikos, G.K., Garzonis, S., Paleologue, A., Bousvaros, G.A. & Papadovannakis, N. (1959) Benign myalgic encephalomyelitis. An outbreak in a Nurses' School in Athens. *Lancet*, **1**, 693–696

Dillon, M.J., Marshall, W.C., Dudgeon, J.A. & Steigman, A.J. (1974) Epidemic Neuromyasthenia: outbreak among nurses at a children's hospital. *British Medical Journal*, **1**, 301–305

Dubois, R.E., Seeley, J.K., Brus, I., Sakamoto, K., Ballow, M., Harada, S., Bechtold, T.A., Pearson, G. & Portilo, D.T. (1984) Chronic Mononucleosis Syndrome. *Southern Medical Journal*, **77**, 1376–1382

Fegan, K.G., Behan, P.O. & Bell, E.J. (1983) Myalgic Encephalomyelitis: report of an epidemic. *Journal of the Royal College of General Practitioners*, **33**, 335–337

Friman, G., Schiller, H.H. & Schwartz, M.S. (1977) Disturbed neuromuscular transmission in viral infections. *Scandinavian Journal of Infectious Diseases*, **9**, 99–103

Gadian, D., Radda, G.K., Ross, B., Hockaday, J., Bore, P., Taylor, D. & Syles, P. (1981) PNMR examination of a myopathy. *Lancet*, **2**, 775

Galpine, J.F. & Brady, C. (1957) Benign myalgic encephalomyelitis. *Lancet*, **1**, 757–758

Gilliam, A.G. (1938) Epidemiological study of an epidemic diagnosed as poliomyelitis occurring among the personnel of the Los Angeles County General Hospital during the summer of 1934. Public Health Bulletin No. 240 – April 1938. United States Public Health Service, Washington, D.C.: Government Printing Office

Gsell, O. (1938) *Abortive Poliomyelitis*. Leipzig: Verlag Thieme

Gsell, O. (1949) Abortive Poliomyelitis. *Helvetica Medica Acta*, **16**, 170–172

Hamblin, T.J., Hussain, J., Akbar, A.N., Tank, Y.C., Smith, J.L. & Jones, D.B. (1983) Immunological reason for chronic ill-health after infectious mononucleosis. *British Medical Journal*, **287**, 85–89

Hardtke, E.F. (1955) Iceland Disease in Indiana. *Journal of the Indiana State Medical Association*, **48**, 245–250

Hart, T.M. & Luck, J.V. (1934) Orthopedic aspects of Los Angeles County 1934 poliomyelitis epidemic. *American Journal of Public Health*, **24**, 1224–1228

Henderson, D.A. & Shelokov, A. (1959) Epidemic Neuromyasthenia – Clinical Syndrome? *New England Journal of Medicine*, **260**, 757–764, 814–818

Hill, R.C.J., Cheetham, R.W.S. & Wallace, H. (1959) Epidemic Myalgic Encephalomyelopathy. The Durban outbreak. *Lancet*, **1**, 689–693

Hoagland, R.J. (1955) The transmission of infectious mononucleosis. *American Journal of Medical Science*, **229**, 262–272

Innes, S.G.B. (1970) Encephalomyelitis resembling benign myalgic encephalomyelitis. *Lancet*, **1**, 969–971

Inoue, Y.K. & Nishibe, Y. (1973) Serological relationship between SMON virus and avian laryngotracheitis virus. *Lancet*, **1**, 776–777

Inoue, Y.K., Nishibe, Y. & Kimura, T. (1971) Virus associated with SMON in Japan. *Lancet*, **1**, 853–854

Jamal, G.A. & Hansen, S. (1985) Electrophysiological studies in the post viral fatigue syndrome. *Journal of Neurology, Neurosurgery and Psychiatry*, **48**, 691–694

Jellinek, J.E. (1956) Benign Encephalomyelitis. *Lancet*, **2**, 494–495

Jones, J.P., Ray, G., Minnich, L.L., Hocks, M.J., Kiblet, R. & Incas, D.O. (1985) Evidence for active Epstein-Barr virus infection in patients with persistent unexplained illnesses: elevated early

antigen antibodies. *Annals of Internal Medicine*, **201**, 1–7

Keighley, B.D. & Bell, E.J. (1983) Sporadic myalgic encephalomyelitis in a rural practice. *Journal of the Royal College of General Practitioners*, **33**, 339–341

Kendell, R.E. (1967) The psychiatric sequelae of Benign Myalgic Encephalomyelitis. *British Journal of Psychiatry*, **113**, 833–840

Leading article. (1955) Infectious Mononucleosis. *British Medical Journal*, **2**, 309–310

Leading article. (1956) A New Clinical Entity? *Lancet*, **1**, 789–790

Leading article. (1967) Coxsackie B5 virus infections during 1965. *British Medical Journal*, **4**, 575–577

Leading article. (1978) Epidemic Myalgic Encephalomyelitis. *British Medical Journal*, **1**, 1436–1437

Leading article. (1985) E.B.V. and Persistent Malaise. *Lancet*, **1**, 1017–1018

Lyle, W.H. (1959) An outbreak of disease believed to have been caused by ECHO 9 virus. *Annals of Internal Medicine*, **51**, 248–269

Lyle, W.H. & Chamberlain, R.N., eds. (1978) Epidemic Neuromyasthenia 1934–1977. Current approaches. *Postgraduate Medical Journal*, **54**, 705–774

Macrae, A.D. & Galpine, J.F. (1954) An illness resembling poliomyelitis observed in nurses. *Lancet*, **2**, 350–352

Marinacci, A.A. & Von Hagen, K.C. (1965) The value of the electromyogram in the diagnosis of Iceland Disease. *Bulletin of the Los Angeles Neurological Society*, **30**, 161–168

McEvedy, C.P. & Beard, A.W. (1970a) Royal Free epidemic of 1955: a reconsideration. *British Medical Journal*, **1**, 7–11

McEvedy, C.P. & Beard, A.W. (1970b) Concept of Benign Myalgic Encephalomyelitis. *British Medical Journal*, **1**, 11–15

McEvedy, C.P., Griffith, A. & Hall, T. (1966) Two School Epidemics. *British Medical Journal*, **2**, 1300

Medical staff of the Royal Free Hospital (1957) An outbreak of encephalomyelitis in the Royal Free Hospital Group, London in 1955. *British Medical Journal*, **2**, 895–904

Melnick, J.L., Wang, S., Seidel, E., Muchinik, G., Zhand, L. & Lanford, R.E. (1984) Characterisation of IM virus which is frequently isolated from cerebrospinal fluid of patients with Multiple Sclerosis and other chronic diseases of the central nervous system. *Journal of Virology*, **52**, 739–744

Miller, H.G., Stanton, J.B. & Gibbons, J.L. (1956) Parainfectious encephalomyelitis and related syndromes. A critical review of neurological complications of certain specific fevers. *Quarterly Journal of Medicine*, **25**, 427

Moss, P.D. & McEvedy, C.P. (1966) An epidemic of overbreathing among schoolgirls. *British Medical Journal*, **2**, 1295–1300

Okuda, K., Takedatsu, H., Shingo, M., Matsuura, D., Urakawa, S. & Emura, T. (1965) *Brain and Nerve (Tokyo)*, **17**, 895

Pampiglione, G., Harris, R. & Kennedy, J. (1978) Electro-encephalographic investigations in myalgic encephalomyelitis. *Postgraduate Medical Journal*, **54**, 752

Pappenheimer, A.M., Bailey, O.T., Cheever, F.S. & Daniels, J.B. (1951) Experimental polyradiculitis in monkeys. *Journal of Neuropathology and Clinical Neurology*, **1**, 48–62

Parish, J.G. (1974) Epidemic Neuromyasthenia: a reappraisal. *IRCS Journal of International Research Communications (Medical Science)*, **2**, 22–26

Parish, J.G. (1978) Early outbreaks of 'epidemic neuromyasthenia'. *Postgraduate Medical Journal*, **54**, 711

Pellew, R.A.A. (1951) A clinical description of a disease resembling poliomyelitis seen in Adelaide 1949–51. *Medical Journal of Australia*, **1**, 944–946

Pellew, R.A.A. & Miles, J.A.R. (1955) Further investigations on a disease resembling poliomyelitis seen in Adelaide. *Medical Journal of Australia*, **42**, 480–482

Poskanzer, D.C. (1970) Epidemic malaise. *British Medical Journal*, **2**, 420–421

Poskanzer, D.C., Henderson, D.A., Kunkle, E.C., Kalter, S.S., Clement, W.M. & Bond, J.O. (1957) Epidemic Neuromyasthenia. An outbreak in Punta Gorda, Florida. *New England Journal of Medicine*, **257**, 356–364

Ramsay, A.M. (1978) Epidemic Neuro-myasthenia 1955–1978. *Postgraduate Medical Journal*, **54**, 718

Ramsay, A.M. (1957) Encephalomyelitis simulating poliomyelitis and hysteria. *Lancet*, **2**, 1196–1200

Ramsay, A.M. & O'Sullivan, E. (1956) Encephalomyelitis simulating polio-myelitis. *Lancet*, **1**, 761–766

Ramsay, A.M. & Rundle, A. (1979) Clinical and biochemical findings in ten patients with benign myalgic encephalo-myelitis. *Postgraduate Medical Journal*, **55**, 856–857

Richardson, A.T. (1956) Some aspects of the Royal Free Hospital epidemic. *Annals of Physical Medicine*, **3**, 81–89

Scott, B.D. (1970) Epidemic Malaise. *British Medical Journal*, **1**, 170

Scott, T.F.M. (1967) Post-infectious and vaccinial encephalitis. *Medical Clinics of North America*, **51**, 701

Shelokov, A., Habel, K., Verder, E. & Welsh, W. (1957) Epidemic Neuro-myasthenia. An outbreak of poliomyelitis-like illness in student nurses. *New England Journal of Medicine*, **257**, 345–355

Shumate, J.B., Katnik, R., Ruiz, M., Kaiser, K., Brooke, M.H. & Carroll, J.R. (1979) Myoadenylate deaminase deficiency. *Muscle and Nerve*, **2**, 213–216

Sigurdsson, B. & Gudmundsson, K.G. (1956) Clinical findings six years after outbreak of Akureyri Disease. *Lancet*, **1**, 766–767

Sigurdsson, B., Gudnadottir, M. & Petursson, G. (1958) Response to poliomyelitis vaccination. *Lancet*, **1**, 370–371

Sigurdsson, B., Sigurjonsson, J., Sigurdsson, J.H.J., Thorkelsson, J. & Gudmundsson, K.G. (1950) A disease epidemic in Iceland simulating polio-myelitis. *American Journal of Hygiene*, **52**, 222

Sotomayer, L. (1969) *Epidemic Diencephalitis*. New York: Pageant Press

Southern, P. & Oldstone, M.B.A. (1986) Medical consequences of persistent viral infections. *New England Journal of Medicine*, **314**, 359–367

Straus, S.E., Tosato, G. & Armstrong, G. (1985) Persisting illness and fatigue in adults with evidence of Epstein-Barr virus infection. *Annals of Internal Medicine*, **102**, 7–18

Tilzey, A.J., Signy, M. & Banatvala, J.E. (1986) (Letter) *Lancet*, **1**, 1492

Tobi, M. & Morag, A. (1984) Chronic Mononucleosis. In *Immune Deficiency and Cancer*. Edited by D. Purtilo. pp.349–366. New York and London: Plenum Medical.

Tobi, M., Morag, A., Ravid, Z., Chowers, I., Feldman-Weiss, V., Michaeli, Y., Ben-Chetrit, E., Shalit, M. & Knobler, H. (1982) Prolonged atypical illness associated with serological evidence of persistent Epstein-Barr virus infection. *Lancet*, **1**, 61–64

Wallis, A.L. (1955) An unusual epidemic. *Lancet*, **2**, 290

Wallis, A.L. (1957) An investigation into an unusual disease seen in epidemic and sporadic form in a general practice in Cumberland in 1955 and subsequent years. M.D. Thesis, Edinburgh University

White, D.N. & Burtch, R.B. (1954)
Iceland Disease – a new infection
simulating acute anterior poliomyelitis.
*Neurology*, **4**, 506–516

Wilkinson, J.H. (1978) Clinical
neurology. *Journal of the Royal Society
of Medicine*, **71**, 241

Wilson, J.C. & Walker, P.J. (1936) Acute
anterior poliomyelitis: orthopaedic
aspects of California epidemic of 1934.
*Archives of Internal Medicine*, **57**,
477–491